CW01625405

Case Presentations in
Obstetrics and Gynaec

Other published titles

Case Presentations in Clinical Geriatric Medicine
Case Presentations in Endocrinology and Diabetes
Case Presentations in Gastrointestinal Disease
Case Presentations in General Surgery
Case Presentations in Heart Disease
Case Presentations in Neurology
Case Presentations in Paediatrics
Case Presentations in Renal Medicine
Case Presentations in Respiratory Medicine
Case Presentations in Urology

Case Presentations in Obstetrics and Gynaecology

T. Ian Wagstaff, BSc, MD, BS, FRCOG
Consultant Obstetrician and Gynaecologist, Newcastle General Hospital
Clinical Lecturer, University of Newcastle

BUTTERWORTH
HEINEMANN

Butterworth-Heinemann Ltd
Linacre House, Jordan Hill, Oxford OX2 8DP

A member of the Reed Elsevier group

OXFORD LONDON BOSTON
MUNICH NEW DELHI SINGAPORE SYDNEY
TOKYO TORONTO WELLINGTON

First published 1991
Reprinted 1993

British Library Cataloguing in Publication Data
Wagstaff, T. Ian
Case presentations in obstetrics and gynaecology
1. Gynaecology and obstetrics
I. Title
618

ISBN 0 7506 1189 8

Library of Congress Cataloging in Publication Data
Wagstaff, T. Ian (Thomas Ian)
Case presentations in obstetrics and gynaecology/T. Ian Wagstaff
p. cm.
Includes bibliographical references and index
ISBN 0 7506 1189 8
1. Gynaecology – case studies. 2. Obstetrics – case studies.
3. Gynaecology – examinations, questions, etc. 4. Obstetrics – examinations, questions, etc. I. Title
RG106.W44 1991
618—dc20 90–15148
CIP

Printed and bound in Great Britain by
Biddles Ltd, Guildford and King's Lynn

Preface

The previous books in this series have been addressed to candidates preparing themselves for the MRCP(UK) part 11 examination and in particular to the solution of the 'grey cases' in the written paper. Such questions are not a feature of the higher examinations set by the Royal College of Obstetricians and Gynaecologists, but the format of the series is ideally suited for those doctors preparing themselves for the clinical component of this College's Membership examination (MRCOG).

This handbook is not intended to be a comprehensive textbook of obstetrics and gynaecology nor on its own a complete revision text. Its purpose is to assist the candidate to prepare for the clinical examination and the ensuing viva.

Each presentation consists of a case history presented together with the salient findings on physical examination. Questions are posed regarding further management and investigation. The cases are original, but reflect those that have been presented to our own junior staff in their examinations. The questions asked and the topics discussed mirror their experience. A discussion encompasses the options for management and explores areas of controversy illustrated by the case. A comment alerts the candidate to the examiner's approach in asking the questions and a short bibliography suggests some key references. Where relevant, the outcome of the case is described.

The approach of the book should also be useful for candidates preparing for the DRCOG or similar qualifications outside the United Kingdom.

In a text of this length it is impossible to describe every case that a candidate might encounter, and the cases selected do not necessarily reflect the frequency of pathology in clinical practice. Where the diagnosis is obscure or the case unusual, it is explored in a logical and systematic manner. It is this basically practical approach that is expected of candidates in the examination.

In the text the candidate is referred to as 'he'. This reflects merely convention and does not represent any bias, either against or for the women doctors who present themselves for the examination.

I would like to acknowledge the contributions, help and advice received from Mr S. L. Barron, Mr P. Hilton, Dr E. V. M. McGoogan and Mr E. J. Thomas and also the support of Dr C. A. Snodgrass, Mr A. S. McIntosh and Mr M. M. Singh, my colleagues at Newcastle General Hospital. I am grateful to Sylvia Hull of Butterworths who offered me the challenge to write this book and to Lucy Sayer who supervised the confinement. Finally, I would like to thank my long suffering secretary Mrs Debbie Slaney whose patience with the writer appears to be limitless.

Dedicated to Thomas C. Wagstaff and Elsie Wagstaff

Contents

Abbreviations

AC	Abdominal circumference
AFP	Alpha feto-protein
AIHA	Autoimmune haemolytic anaemia
APH	Antepartum haemorrhage
APTT	Activated partial thromboplastin time
ARM	Artificial rupture of membranes
AST	Aspartate amino-transferase
BP	Blood pressure
BPD	Biparietal diameter
BSO	Bilateral salpingo-oophorectomy
CHB	Congenital heart block
CNS	Central nervous system
CRL	Crown-rump length
CSF	Cerebrospinal fluid
CT	Computerised tomography
CTG	Cardiotochograph
CVP	Central venous pressure
CXR	Chest x-ray
DIC	Disseminated intravascular coagulation
EDD	Expected date of delivery
EUA	Examination under anaesthetic
FAI	Free androgen index
FDPs	Fibrin degradation products
FL	Femur length
FSH	Follicular stimulating hormone
FTA-abs	Absorbed fluorescent Treponema antibody test
HC	Head circumference
IGT	Impaired glucose tolerance
IHCP	Intrahepatic cholestasis of pregnancy
ITP	Immune thrombocytopenia
IUCD	Intrauterine contraceptive device
IUGR	Intrauterine growth retardation
IVU	Intravenous urogram
JVP	Jugular venous pressure

KCCT	Kaolin cephalin clotting time
LDH	Lactic acid dehydrogenase
LH	Luteinising hormone
LLETZ	Large loop excision of the transformation zone
LMP	Last menstrual period
LOT	Left occipito-transverse position
L-S Ratio	Lecithin sphingomyelin ratio
MAP	Mean arterial pressure
MCH	Mean corpuscular haemoglobin
MCHC	Mean corpuscular haemoglobin concentration
MCV	Mean corpuscular volume
MSU	Midstream specimen of urine
NMR	Nuclear magnetic resonance
OD	Optical density
OGTT	Oral glucose tolerance test
PCOS	Polycystic ovarian syndrome
PMS	Premenstrual syndrome
PPF	Plasma protein fraction
RDS	Respiratory distress syndrome
SGA	Small for gestation age
SHBG	Sex hormone binding globulin
SLE	Systemic lupus erythematosus
TAH	Total abdominal hysterectomy
TPHA	Treponema pallidum haemagglutination assay
UPP	Urethral pressure profile
VCU	Videocystourethrogram
VDRL	Venereal disease reference laboratory

The clinical examination

In the sense that this part of the examination reflects the daily experience of the candidate, it should present little difficulty. The fact that approximately 45% of candidates fail this part is therefore surprising. It is particularly ironic that candidates should stumble at this final hurdle because under current regulations, only those candidates with a prospect of passing the whole examination are allowed to sit the clinical component. Myths abound as to why candidates have failed. Too often the reason was simply that the examinees abandoned their usual practice in an effort to impress the examiners, or read into the straightforward questions complexities that were not present.

Introduction

Candidates are allocated one obstetrical and one gynaecological case. They have 45 minutes in which to obtain the histories and to examine the patients. On occasion an examiner may be present at this phase of the examination. Candidates are sometimes asked to defer the abdominal examination of the obstetric case until the examiners are present. A vaginal examination of the gynaecological case should be performed only when requested by the examiners and in their presence. After the allotted time has elapsed the examiners meet the candidate, usually at the bedside, to listen to the case histories and to observe the candidate undertaking any clinical examination they request. Discussion of the cases and their management usually takes place away from the patients in another room.

Points to note

The details of the clinical examination sent to candidates include instructions on how to travel to the hospital concerned. A generous margin of time should be allowed for any arrangements, especially when travelling by public transport. Time before the examination should be spent thinking about those items to be included in any history and the technique to demonstrate the clinical examination. The candidate should be suitably dressed for a 'professional' examination and free of any impedimenta such as jewellery or long hair that might interfere with the efficient performance of a clinical examination. A clean white coat is quite acceptable. The hands should be clean and the nails trimmed. A neat and tidy appearance will encourage the patient to respond positively to the candidate, thus assisting in the recording of a comprehensive history.

All necessary instruments are usually provided but candidates are advised to carry their own stethoscopes, tape measures, obstetric calculator and two pens.

Members of the hospital staff direct candidates to their allotted patients. This is the time to establish whether there are any restrictions to the physical examination. The candidate should also enquire if there are any specimens of urine to test. Such testing is usually by 'dipsticks'. Occasionally facilities are provided to microscope the urine, but in such cases, the history is usually very relevant. If no specimen is available enquire if the urine is known to contain any abnormal constituents.

Five minutes should be set aside before the examiners arrive to identify the essential points of the history and examination. A differential diagnosis should be established where necessary and a proposed plan for the patient's subsequent care worked out. If a good history has been obtained then with a little reflection many of the examiner's questions can be anticipated.

Too often the presentation of the history is long winded and repetitive. It is in the candidate's interest to save as much time as possible in the actual presentation of the cases. The examiner wishes to explore the candidate's knowledge rather than his ignorance and if difficulties are to be encountered in the viva then the more time available to move on to another topic the better. It is good policy to complete the history with a succinct summary of the essential points. The presentation will be much more impressive if the history can be given clearly and logically without constant referral to notes. Such a presentation shows the examiner that the candidate can obtain all the information required and at the same time assimilate and evaluate it.

A detailed account of the clinical examination is beyond the remit of this book but a few comments may help. The examiners insist that the patients be afforded at all times the utmost respect and consideration. Politeness and gentleness coupled with a calm and *purposeful* examination will obtain the best results for the candidate. Addressing the patient by her first name may be fashionable but is not advised. Nursing assistance is usually available and should be recruited when positioning the patient for examination. Exposure of the patient should be adequate, but with concern for modesty. Her agreement should be solicited before proceeding and at the conclusion of the examination the patient should be made comfortable, covered and thanked.

The positioning of the patient for gynaecological examination is a matter of personal taste and the candidate is strongly advised to adopt the technique with which he is most familiar. The candidate may be asked to explain his preference for the chosen technique.

The clinical examination concludes with a discussion of the case. The candidate must *listen carefully* to the questions. The examiners usually will ask for the candidate's opinion and management of the case. There may be several options, in which case they are looking for a commitment by the candidate to a particular line of action. They will not welcome a review of the literature no matter how eminent the authorities. The examination is a prelude to senior clinical practice and it is the candidate's clinical ability that is being assessed not a knowledge of the literature. An examiner may adopt an alternative stance during the discussion, in which case, the candidate will be expected to provide valid reasons to support his own opinion. Few opinions in medicine are absolute and providing the candidate can substantiate his approach, and it is reasonable, then he will not be penalized. A second examiner is always present to ensure fair play.

The best preparation for the clinical examination is PRACTICE and after that MORE PRACTICE ideally under examination conditions. Most consultants are only too happy to provide this kind of supervision. No matter how knowledgeable a candidate may be, failure will result if he is unable to demonstrate the basic clinical skills or the ability to deduce from the evidence at his disposal an acceptable and safe policy of management. Having completed the training required for the MRCOG it is extremely unlikely that any candidate will lack the knowledge to pass this component of the examination.

Case presentations

Case 1

The 30-year-old primigravida presented in the antenatal clinic with a history of 12 weeks amenorrhoea. There was no significant family or previous medical history. Her general examination was satisfactory with a booking blood pressure of 110/70 mmHg. The uterus was considered marginally large for dates. Urinalysis was normal. Her blood group was A Rhesus positive.

By 18 weeks the symphysial-fundal measurement was 22 cm. Ultrasound confirmed a twin pregnancy. Twin 1 had a biparietal diameter (BPD) of 4.4 cm and twin 2 a BPD of 4.0 cm. There were no apparent fetal abnormalities.

The patient was booked for hospital care and arrangements made to see her fortnightly to 28 weeks and weekly thereafter. Folate supplements and oral iron were prescribed.

At 28 weeks the fundal height was 34 cm and on palpation there appeared to be excess amniotic fluid. This was confirmed on ultrasound. The BPD of twin 1 was 7.5 cm and twin 2, 7.0 cm. No antibodies were detected in the maternal blood.

Four weeks later the patient's blood pressure was 140/90 mmHg. There was pitting oedema to midshin but urinalysis remained normal. The fundus was now at the xiphisternum and the fetal parts were barely palpable. The patient was complaining of considerable discomfort and an inability to sustain her usual activities. She was admitted to hospital.

On ultrasound, the BPD of twin 1 was 8.3 cm. The head circumference (HC) was 31 cm and the abdominal circumference (AC) 30 cm. The equivalent measurements for twin 2 were BPD 7.4 cm, HC 26.5 cm and AC 21 cm. Gross polyhydramnios was confirmed and detailed scanning failed to identify any fetal abnormalities.

A maternal fasting blood sugar level was 3.9 mmol/l and a 2-h postprandial blood sugar level was 4.3 mmol/l.

By 36 weeks the patient's blood pressure was averaging 150/100 mmHg and routine urinalysis revealed ++ albumin (Albustix). A 24-h urine collection contained 900 mg of protein. Urea and electrolytes were normal. The plasma urate level was 0.42 μmol/l and the creatinine clearance 115 ml/min. The daily fetal heart traces for each twin were consistently scored between 8–10 on the Fischer rating. The ultrasound findings were: twin 1, cephalic, BPD 8.6 cm, HC 30 cm, AC 29.2 cm; twin 2 breech, BPD 7.5 cm, HC 27 cm, AC 21.5 cm.

Questions

Summarize the obstetric problem described

This is a primigravid patient with a twin pregnancy at 36 weeks gestation. She has developed polyhydramnios and pre-eclampsia. The second twin presents by the breech and on ultrasound criteria suffers from asymmetrical growth retardation.

Explain how you might manage this case.

At this gestation with pre-eclampsia and the second twin showing signs of intrauterine growth retardation delivery must be considered. Delay runs the risk of the mother developing eclampsia or the smaller baby dying *in utero*. On the other hand, at this gestation the babies pose a problem for neonatal care. If suitable facilities are not immediately available then intrauterine transfer to a regional unit should be arranged before the maternal condition contraindicates such a transfer. If the maternal condition does deteriorate, then delivery on site would be necessary, with a paediatric flying squad either in attendance or prepared to collect the baby(s) should the need arise. The pre-eclampsia is of a moderate degree and providing that the maternal condition remained stable in terms of blood pressure, freedom from symptoms and acceptable blood chemistry, then it would be possible to try for a little more time in the interest of fetal maturity. Fetal well-being would be assessed by daily cardiotocography and if possible by more sophisticated techniques such as the measurement of biophysical profiles and umbilical artery end diastolic flow. It would be unwise to delay beyond the 38th week. The second twin presents by the breech and appears growth retarded. Second born twins are more likely to die from intrapartum anoxia and perinatal asphyxia and this baby would be particularly vulnerable. Delivery should therefore be by caesarean section. The reason for the growth retardation in the single twin is unknown and in the presence of polyhydramnios it is possible that this reflects some fetal abnormality but the detailed examinations performed in pregnancy failed to demonstrate any anomaly. This concern must be explored with the parents.

Is polyhydramnios commoner in monozygotic or dizygotic twins?

Although commoner in twin than in singleton pregnancies it is probably no commoner in monozygos than in dizygos twins.

What feature of monochorionic twins is associated with twins of significantly differing birthweight?

The feto-fetal transfusion syndrome or twin transfusion syndrome.

Discussion

The mother was delivered of the twins by caesarean section, under epidural anaesthesia, at 37 weeks. The hydramnios was associated with twin 1, a male weighing 2400 g, which was plethoric in appearance. Despite breathing normally in air he remained peripherally cyanosed. Twin 2, also male, weighed 1825 g and was extremely pale. Resuscitation was straight forward but the baby soon required dextrose infusion for the correction of hypoglycaemia. The placenta was monochorionic and diamniotic. The two thirds of the placenta associated with twin 2 was swollen and oedematous, the remainder appeared congested.

The appearances were consistent with the feto-fetal transfusion syndrome. This diagnosis should be suspected if the weight of one of like sex twins is less than 80% of its partner. Such discrepancies can occur in discordant twins because of local factors, e.g. retroplacental bleeding, infarction, poor placentation etc. The diagnosis is established by examination of the fetal venous blood. A blood haemoglobin difference of more than 5 g/dl between twin members is significant. In the case described, twin 1 had a haemoglobin concentration of 27.6 g/dl with a haematocrit of 0.88, and twin 2 a haemoglobin concentration of 14.8 g/dl and a haematocrit of 0.44. The twins were consanguineous for 10 blood groups.

The cause lies in the placenta. In monochorionic placentae it is common to identify on the surface, connections between vessels derived from each fetus. These are usually artery to artery. Deeper connections occur at capillary level within the placental cotyledons. The potential exists for one twin to 'exsanguinate' into the other. The factors determining the onset and rate of transfusion are unknown. As in this case transfusion may take place over a long period during pregnancy. The placenta of the donor twin is disproportionately large, the villi oedematous and the trophoblast hypertrophied. The small villous capillaries contain immature nucleated red cells. Despite its size, the donor placenta is inefficient and intrauterine growth retardation is common. The discrepancy between the levels of maternally derived IgG in donor and recipient is greater than for other proteins, e.g. total protein, albumin, transferrin and alpha-1-antitrypsin, suggesting impaired trophoblastic function in the donor. The recipient placenta is smaller but the trophoblast is thinned and the capillaries engorged with red cells. Because of the increased blood viscosity cardiac hypertrophy may be present in the recipient. The recipient's renal glomeruli are frequently dilated and appear more mature than the period of gestation would suggest. This configuration may contribute to the common observation of polyhydramnios in the recipient's sac. Likewise the relative hyperproteinaemia of the recipient by altering the osmotic equilibrium could draw more water from the maternal compartment.

Twin to twin transfusion can occur acutely during parturition through the large superficial anastomoses. Twins of like sex and similar birthweight then exhibit the phenomena of anaemia and hypovolaemia in the donor and polycythaemia and overload in the recipient. However, pallor and hypovolaemia in one twin can result from a fetomaternal haemorrhage in which case fetal cells will be detected in the maternal circulation by a Kleihauer estimation.

It is the recipient twin that generally demands the more urgent management at birth. Polycythaemia may lead to cerebral irritation, convulsions and cause cerebral and other vascular thromboses. The increased blood viscosity may precipitate heart failure. Venesection may cause problems with hypovolaemia before the haematocrit is reduced. The treatment of choice is partial exchange transfusion to reduce the haematocrit to approximately 60% using fresh frozen plasma.

The donor, if small for dates, may require glucose for hypoglycaemia. Usually during pregnancy transfusion has occurred slowly enough for compensation in terms of blood volume to take place. The donor may show signs of high output failure or respiratory difficulties in which case exchange transfusion with packed cells to correct the red cell imbalance is indicated.

Feto-fetal transfusion syndrome may cause the death of one fetus *in utero*. It has been estimated that 15% of all monochorial twin pregnancies are affected by the syndrome contributing to the higher fetal loss in such twins.

Further reading

GALEA, P., SCOTT, J. M. and GOEL, K. M. (1982) Feto-fetal transfusion syndrome. *Archives of Disease in Childhood*, **57**, 781–794

MacGILLIVARY, I., NIJLANDER, P. P. S. and CORNEY, G. (1975) *Human Multiple Reproduction*, W. B. Saunders, London

Case 2

The patient was a 48-year-old Polish emigré resident in the UK for 17 months. She was a widow. For 12 months she had experienced increasing dyspnoea on moderate exertion causing her to pause in her activities and catch her breath. She had also complained of some left-sided chest pain particularly associated with exertion but not typical of angina pectoris. She lived with her daughter. Their circumstances were adequate and she enjoyed a balanced diet. She was referred in the first instance to the cardiologist who ruled out any cardiac abnormality but confirmed an iron deficiency anaemia. She denied any untoward blood loss and in particular assured the physician that her periods were unremarkable.

Her general examination was normal apart from pallor and a soft systolic ejection murmur attributed to anaemia. She was well nourished weighing 58.8 kg, and was 160 cm tall.

Her haemoglobin was 7.8 g/dl. The MCV was 64 fl. The reticulocyte count was 2%. Haemoglobin electrophoresis was normal. Stool occult blood tests had been negative on three occasions. Her serum iron was 3.5 μmol/l. A clotting screen was normal and she was euthyroid according to her thyroid function tests. A chest x-ray was normal and urinalysis confirmed the absence of haematuria and infection. Her serum electrolytes were normal, she was not jaundiced clinically or biochemically and her liver function tests were normal.

On the completion of these investigations she was placed on oral iron for two months after which her haemoglobin rose to 13.3 g/dl with an MCV of 86 fl.

Because the cause of the anaemia had not been explained the physician questioned her again about the menstrual pattern. She explained that she had been too embarrassed to discuss such matters before. She described that her menarche had been at 13 years of age and her cycle had always been regular, 26–28 days, although the duration of the periods had increased over the time in question from 3 to 7 days. The loss on days 2 and 3 were the heaviest requiring the frequent changing of two sanitary pads at a time and the necessity to rise during the night to change. The periods were accompanied by mild abdominal discomfort such as she always had; there had been no recognizable change from this point of view. There was no inter or postcoital bleeding.

In the gynaecological clinic the normal general examination was confirmed. A pelvic examination was entirely normal. The uterus was of normal size, anteverted and mobile. There was no adnexal pathology.

She was admitted to the hospital for premenstrual hysteroscopy and curettage. The normal clinical findings were confirmed. Hysteroscopy revealed a normal uterine cavity. The histological examination of the curettings was reported as showing normal secretory endometrium with no atypia.

When seen for follow-up 3 months later the patient reported that she had no further periods and that she felt very well. The gynaecologist reassured her that all had been normal at her operation and that it was possible that she was approaching the menopause. She was discharged from the clinic.

Three months later she was referred back by her GP. After her last visit she had not had any bleeding for 2 months. She then experienced a very heavy vaginal loss that had persisted unstopped for 2 weeks. There was then a break of 3 days before the bleeding recommenced, albeit much lighter, for a further 2 weeks and was continuing. An urgent haemoglobin estimation was reported as 8.3 g/dl. The findings on examination were unchanged. She was admitted to hospital and received tablets that curtailed the loss.

Questions

How would you account for this series of events?

The patient presented with the history of menorrhagia, i.e. excessive regular menstruation. She was investigated thoroughly by the physicians who excluded the usual medical causes for excessive menstruation. The hysteroscopy and curettage in turn excluded local pelvic pathology as a cause of the excessive menses. The identification of secretory changes in the endometrium confirmed ovulation taking place in that cycle. The diagnosis at this point was dysfunctional uterine bleeding. When seen for review there had been 3 months amenorrhoea. Two weeks later she proceeded to bleed heavily and although this lightened it has persisted to the present. The patient is now 48-years-old and approaching the menopause.

In this phase of reproductive life anovulatory cycles can supervene. The absence of ovulation results in a prolonged proliferative phase under the influence of oestrogen unmodified by progesterone from a corpus luteum. Eventually the hormonal support fails and prolonged and very heavy bleeding can result.

This pattern of bleeding is sometimes referred to as metropathia haemorrhagica and is associated with cystic glandular hyperplasia in the endometrium. A follicular cyst is often felt in the adnexum.

This patient is widowed and not apparently sexually active. Had this not been the case there would be the possibility of an early pregnancy complication although the unchanged physical findings and her age would make this unlikely.

How are you going to manage this case now?

The first priority is to control the bleeding which has already made her anaemic. She should be admitted to hospital for blood transfusion. The pattern of bleeding is likely to persist and prophylactic treatment with iron will not restore the situation rapidly enough to cope with any further insult. Blood would be administered best as packed cells to avoid overloading the circulation and precipitating congestive cardiac failure.

Two options are available to curtail the bleeding. Progesterone can be given by injection or orally (norethisterone 10 mg three times daily). This can be given for two to three weeks during which the hyperplastic endometrium will be converted into the secretory phase and withdrawal of the preparation will initiate a normal shedding of the endometrium. In this specific case there would seem to be little value at this age in allowing her to resume a natural cycle which has already made her anaemic and the risk is also of another precipitate anovulatory bleed. After transfusion and control of the loss with progestogen, I would proceed to an abdominal hysterectomy. A second option would be to use oestrogen to curtail the bleeding by further promoting proliferation of the endometrium. With the withdrawal of this stimulus further heavy bleeding can be anticipated but to provide a short interval before hysterectomy this treatment is a possibility. Unfortunately large doses of oestrogen are often necessary (0.1 mg ethinyloestradiol 4-hourly) and high doses of oestrogen are not advisable before surgery for fear of embolic complications. Progesterone is the preferred option.

This patient is 48 years of age and the onset of anovulatory cycles might in fact herald the onset of the menopause. Why not continue with her hormonal therapy on a cyclical basis?

The onset of the menopause is variable. On average it is at the age of 51 years but in this case it could be much later. Control of the menses with progesterones can be difficult so that the dosage has to be increased and side-effects can be troublesome. This patient has experienced ill-health as a result of her dysfunctional uterine bleeding and surgery would give her the certain relief she requires.

Would you remove the ovaries ?

I would discuss this with the patient first. Ovarian carcinoma is the most frequent cause of death from genital cancer. It is difficult to identify in the early stages and is usually silent until the disease is advanced. There is no accurate technique for screening the population. The result is, that when the disease presents, it is often advanced and irretrievable. With hormone replacement therapy now freely available there is not the same concern as before about the precipitation of menopausal symptoms from oestrogen deficiency in the woman who is still menstruating. Having discussed matters with her, I would leave her to make her own decision, with the proviso that if there is any concern as to the appearances of the ovaries at operation then they would be removed.

Apart from hysterectomy do you know of any other surgical techniques that might be suitable?

There is increasing interest in techniques that ablate the endometrium rendering it unresponsive to hormonal stimuli. Hysteroscopic endometrial ablation with the neodymium-YAG laser and hysteroscopic resection of the endometrium using the urological resectoscope have both been described. These techniques have the advantage of avoiding major abdominal surgery and reducing the patient's recovery period.

I think that I would agree with you that this patient had menorrhagia in that her natural menstrual function rendered her anaemic. This is only rarely the case in young women who attend the clinic complaining of menorrhagia. Is the diagnosis justified in these cases?

Rarely! The upper limit of normal for the monthly menstrual flow has been assessed as 80 ml. This provides an objective point of reference. Unfortunately of a population of patients presenting with 'menorrhagia' only 38% satisfied this criterion. The objective measurement of the menstrual loss is a messy and time consuming business for the doctor and patient alike and thoroughly distasteful.

There is no easy, accurate way of measuring the menstrual loss and management depends on the patient's subjective assessment. As part of the investigation of such cases it is usual to undertake curettage of the uterus. This is a purely diagnostic procedure and yet following it some patients claim improvement and even cure. There is no logic for this and one must assume that the original diagnosis was in error. For the same reason, the efficacy of various medical treatments given in good faith and based on trial data, rarely achieves the expected rates of success.

In a young woman with dysfunctional uterine bleeding what medical treatment can you prescribe?

Examination of the menstrual effluent for prostaglandins in women with proven menorrhagia reveals increased levels of prostaglandin E2 and prostacyclin. These particular prostaglandins induce vasodilatation and inhibit platelet aggregation. The PGE2/PGF2 and prostacylin/thromboxane ratios are raised. This would indicate a disorder of prostaglandin synthesis at the level of the myometrium and the endometrium producing disordered haemostasis. Treatment with anti-prostin non-steroidal anti-inflammatory drugs, e.g. mefenamic acid, flufenamic acid and naproxen can half the menstrual loss in women with true menorrhagia. It is of interest that each drug affects the production of different prostaglandins to different degrees. These drugs can also reduce the uterine cramps that frequently aggravate the picture. A great advantage is that these tablets are only taken at the time of menstruation.

Ethamsylate which probably acts by reducing capillary fragility and inhibiting prostaglandin synthesis and tranexamic acid which promotes fibrin stabilization by inhibiting plasminogen activation and fibrinolysis can both produce a significant reduction in the menstrual flow in true menorrhagia.

Women with menorrhagia have normal oestrogen and progesterone levels and ovulate regularly. Suppression of ovulation by the combined oral contraceptive will in most cases reduce the duration and amount of the blood loss.

Frequently the complaint arises when the patient reverts to her natural cycle having first come off the pill and then having been sterilized. Such patients are reluctant once more to take a drug which many consider to carry a risk for them. The preparations are not suitable for women with cardiovascular risk factors and those over the age of 35 years who smoke.

There is no evidence that supplementary progestogen in the

second half of the cycle improves matters and this drug may in turn produce undesired side-effects.

Danazol 200 mg daily for 3 months appears to reduce the menstrual flow and the improvement tends to persist for a similar period after therapy. Effective non-hormonal contraception is needed where pregnancy is a risk. The preparation is associated with severe side-effects in some cases, e.g. hirsutism, muscle cramps, fluid retention, weight gain and acne. The patients tolerance of the drug is very variable. Unknown is the place of repeated courses of treatment should the problem persist.

From a practical point of view the oral contraceptive is of value in the young woman who also requires contraception. For the older woman whose contraception is secure an anti-prostin, ethamsylate or tranexamic acid should be tried first before resorting to progestogens or danazol with their increased risk of side-effects.

Discussion

Most patients with menorrhagia have no underlying pathology. If objective measurements are made of the menstrual loss then it is apparent that in more than half the patients complaining of excessive loss, the flow is normal. Measurement of the loss quantifies only one aspect of the menses as perceived by the patient. In modern society childbearing is often completed while the mother is relatively young. Because of the financial implications of children, often a sterilization procedure has been performed on one of the partners. The woman's attention is therefore drawn to a natural function that is no longer of any meaning for her. The monthly experience of bleeding, even if unaccompanied by other symptoms, intrudes upon her daily activities at home, at recreation or at work and the natural function becomes the focus of resentment and dissatisfaction. The prospect of prolonged therapy for symptom relief does not appeal. In many cases, the reporting of excessive loss is only a means to the end of ending all menstrual function by removing the uterus. Consequently, there is a mismatch between the incidence of pathology and the frequency with which hysterectomy is carried out, and the degree of this discrepancy is greatest in those countries where the normal is for medical practice to be predominantly in the private sector. In the UK, 20% of women undergo hysterectomy principally for menstrual problems. Often this is a last resort because medical methods have 'failed' but in many cases there was no medical problem and the menstrual function was within normal limits.

The operation itself has a low mortality rate (0.6 per 1000) but there is a significant morbidity. Apart from the immediate common postoperative complications, more severe problems may persist, including bladder and bowel dysfunction. Ill-defined abdominal pain may persist and vault prolapse may subsequently occur. More rarely severe complications such as urinary fistulae can ensue. It has been estimated that menopausal symptoms from oestrogen deficiency may be advanced by as much as 4 years on average. There can be serious psychological sequelae, but these are more likely to occur when the symptom-free patient has been advised to have the operation, e.g. for dysplasia of the cervix or silent carcinoma detected on routine screening. When the patient herself is pushing for the operation she has already recognized the need for the procedure in her own mind and sometimes the operation can actually reduce psychiatric symptoms.

There is however a need for a procedure which will achieve the aim of permanently stopping the periods or grossly reducing the menstrual flow, while avoiding the drawbacks of major surgery. Two techniques are under evaluation.

If the endometrium can be ablated for its full thickness down to the superficial myometrium so that the basal layer and glands are destroyed then even if the hormonal milieu is maintained the epithelium cannot regenerate. Hysteroscopic resection of the endometrium using a high frequency diathermy wire loop passed into the uterus by a urological resectoscope has been successful in providing symptomatic relief in a high proportion of cases. The diathermy wire is used to cut away strips of endometrium from the fundus to the isthmus. The chips of material obtained can be sent for histological evaluation. Areas not resected can be treated by 'roller-ball' electrocoagulation. The technique is relatively quick and can be accomplished as an out-patient procedure. It has been suggested that roller-ball coagulation of the endometrium without resection can give comparable results. The apparatus required is not expensive and is already available in those units where urological surgery is undertaken. One concern is that the uterine cavity is often subsequently obliterated by synechiae. Pockets of endometrium may therefore persist, with the risk of malignant change, which may not manifest itself until the disease is advanced.

An alternative modality is photocoagulation of the endometrium using a neodymium-YAG laser fibre under hysteroscopic control.

The success rate with this treatment has varied between 83% and 96% depending on the experience of the operator and the power of the laser applied within the uterus. The technique is time consuming. The apparatus is expensive and potentially more hazardous to both patient and operators than the CO_2 laser used for cervical ablation. However, the formation of synechiae is reported only infrequently.

Both techniques depend upon constant irrigation of the uterine cavity to wash away debris and blood and at the same time to distend the cavity to facilitate visualization of the endometrium. Large volumes of fluid (dextrose, saline, 32% Dextran 70) are required for irrigation, usually in excess of 10 litres. On average it has been suggested that up to 2 litres may be absorbed into the patient's circulation. The techniques are therefore contraindicated in those patients where circulatory load would constitute a medical problem. Pulmonary oedema is a risk. Unfortunately such patients are often the ones for whom the techniques would be most welcome by avoiding major abdominal procedures. It would seem that the amount of fluid absorbed is unpredictable and idiosyncratic and that a wise precaution might be to conduct the procedure with a central venous pressure line *in situ*. These procedures are not suitable for the enlarged uterus.

It is hoped however that purpose-designed instruments for gynaecological use and improved irrigation systems might solve many of these difficulties.

Endometrial ablation is attractive in its concept and would appear to be effective in providing symptomatic relief in the short term. Long-term follow-up is essential to identify any untoward sequelae for the few in the pursuit of relief for the many.

The role of prophylactic oophorectomy remains controversial and the arguments for and against are strongly expressed by their proponents. A candidate should be prepared to express an opinion which can be reasonably defended. A recent survey reported that in the UK only 24% of gynaecologists are willing to remove the ovaries in women aged 45–49 years. The figure increases to 59% if the woman is premenopausal but over 49 years of age and to 85% if she is menopausal. The arguments for prophylactic oophorectomy centre around the appalling prognosis for ovarian carcinoma, the possibility of ovarian symptomatology developing after surgery and the adequacy of hormone replacement therapy.

The overall 5-year survival rate for ovarian carcinoma is only 25%. Twice as many women die from this condition each year as die from cervical carcinoma where there is an enormous investment in prophylaxis which sometimes results in major surgery for premalignant disease. A figure of 0.2% prospective risk for cancer of the ovary has been quoted for women who have undergone hysterectomy with conservation of the ovaries. On the other hand, it has been calculated that 10% of women who develop ovarian carcinoma would have been saved by prophylactic oophorectomy,a simple technique which would not add to the morbidity of the primary procedure.

The ovaries, if retained, can be the cause of further symptomatology or indeed the persistence of some symptoms that the patient might have considered would be cured by hysterectomy. Posthysterectomy ovarian pain or cyst formation is especially common when the initial procedure was for endometriosis, pelvic inflammatory disease or pelvic pain. Symptoms of the premenstrual syndrome and menstrual migraine may supervene or worsen as the time of ovarian failure approaches. It has been suggested in any case, that on average ovarian failure is advanced by 4 years after hysterectomy and that 34% of women develop ovarian failure or symptoms of the climacteric within 2 years.

There is now good evidence that oestrogen replacement therapy prevents the onset of osteoporosis, reduces the frequency of strokes and heart disease and abolishes most symptoms of the climacteric.

However, the alternative case made is that when the statistical chances for any woman developing ovarian cancer after hysterectomy have been calculated the results reported show enormous variation. These calculations show that the risk of ovarian cancer is less than for all women for a comparable age because ovaries suspected of disease at surgery will have been removed in any case. Persistent pain after hysterectomy indeed may be caused by ovarian factors in some cases but is more likely to be caused by other factors present before hysterectomy but undiagnosed, e.g. irritable bowel syndrome. Not all authorities agree that the evidence is overwhelming that normal ovarian function is not sustained to the normal menopause. If hormone replacement therapy is less than optimal following prophylactic oophorectomy then osteoporosis, hypertension and coronary heart disease are possible sequelae. Hormone replacement therapy is not just a matter of prescribing a few oestrogen pills. The choice of oestrogen and its application need to be tailored to the individual patient's requirement. Supplement with testosterone implants may be necessary to sustain libido.

The final decision on the role of prophylactic oophorectomy is not purely surgical. The patient's view should be the primary consideration after she has had the benefit of a full and informed discussion. The option should not be offered unless the facilities are available to provide and supervise the patient's hormone replacement therapy.

Outcome

The patient was placed on continuous progestogen for 2 weeks during which her bleeding remained suppressed. Transfusion brought her haemoglobin up to 13.2 g/dl. She was admitted for total abdominal hysterectomy. The procedure was uneventful, the pelvic organs were macroscopically normal. The uterus and cervix measured 10 cm in length. The endometrium was soft and bulky with a polypoid configuration. The endometrium was secretory with no atypia. The cervix showed mild reserve cell hyperplasia, there was no dysplasia.

Comment

Gynaecological cases are becoming harder to find for examination purposes and therefore more candidates will find themselves confronted with a case that has a very commonplace history to present and whose examination is absolutely normal. Problems with menstruation constitute the bulk of out-patient referrals. The candidate should seize on the opportunity to demonstrate to the examiner what is in truth his everyday experience. The questions are inevitably straightforward but intended to explore the candidate's understanding of the treatment prescribed. The viva is then a discussion between professionals of the options available and the reasons for selecting a particular course of action for the patient concerned.

Further reading

DAVIES, J. (1989) Hysteroscopic endometrial ablation with the neodymium-YAG laser. *British Journal of Obstetrics and Gynaecology*, **96**, 928–932

DE CHERNEY, A., DIAMOND, M. P., LARY, G. and POLANI, M. L. (1987) Endometrial ablation for intractable uterine bleeding: hysteroscopic resection. *Obstetrics and Gynecology*, **70**, 669–670

MacDONALD, F. (1990) Modern treatment of menorrhagia. *British Journal of Obstetrics and Gynaecology*, **97**, 3–7 (Commentary)

Case 3

The 32-year-old woman presented in her first pregnancy with a history of 10 weeks amenorrhoea. Her cycle was regular (4/28); she had not been taking the oral contraceptive.

Five years earlier she had been the victim of an armed assault. She sustained spinal and abdominal injuries and required a splenectomy and cholecystectomy to control internal haemorrhage. While recovering in a spinal unit she developed a deep vein thrombosis and sustained a pulmonary embolus. She was treated with anticoagulants for a year. On recovery it was apparent that she was left with a profound paraplegia.

She lived with her husband in a specially adapted bungalow and although committed to a wheelchair had succeeded in overcoming her disability to the extent of running her home and leading a varied life in the community.

Chronic constipation was a problem. She took a high fibre diet but still required twice weekly manual evacuation performed by the community nurse. Retention of urine was managed by intermittent self catheterization.

She was not taking any medication.

At booking her blood pressure was 120/70 mmHg. A general and neurological examination confirmed the clinical features of paraplegia consistent with cord transection at the level T9–T10.

At 18 weeks by dates an ultrasound examination had identified a singleton fetus presenting by the breech. The BPD was 4.1 (+/- 0.1) cm. The femoral length was 28 mm, and the configuration of the fetus appeared normal.

Investigations

Initial investigations showed the following:

Blood group: A Rhesus positive
Haemoglobin: 12.6 g/dl, Hct: 0.38,
MCV: 99.6 fl, MCH: 32.9 pg,
MCHC: 33.0 g/dl.
White cell count: 14.1 x 10^9/l,
Granulocytes: 67.9%,
Lymphocytes: 30.1%,
Monocytes: 2.0%.
Platelets: 786 x 10^9/l,
MPV: 7.3 fl,
Pct: 0.574%, Sodium: 133 mmol/l,
Potassium: 4.1 mmol/l,
Chloride: 102 mmol/l,
Bicarbonate: 22 mmol/l,
Anion gap: 13.1 mmol/l,
Urea: 3.2 mmol/l,
Urate: 190 μmol/l,
Creatinine: 70 μmol/l
Creatinine clearance: 140 ml/min
MSU >100 000 *E. coli* per ml
Sensitive to co-trimoxazole, nitrofurantoin, nalidixic acid; resistant to ampicillin.

Questions

What complications of pregnancy do you think might develop in a paraplegic patient?

A major complication of such pregnancies is urinary tract infection. This patient requires repeated self catheterization to avoid urinary retention and an initial culture of the urine grew an *E. coli* resistant to ampicillin. If her renal function were significantly impaired at the onset of pregnancy then termination of pregnancy would have to be considered.

When transection of the cord has occurred above the level of T9–T10 uterine contractions would not be felt by the patient. The onset of labour could be missed with the risk of delivery taking place in unsuitable circumstances. Arrangements might be made to cover delivery towards term, but the problem would be accentuated in the event of pre-term labour. With transection below T11 some sensation might be expected.

Despite the cord transection, normal coordinated uterine contractions develop. However, because of the paresis of the lower abdominal musculature in some patients, coupled with anaesthesia of the pelvic floor, expulsive effort will be minimal and forceps delivery is often required.

Spinal patients require specialized nursing support. This patient requires manual evacuation of the bowel weekly. Nursing in a unit unfamiliar with the management of such patients could result in troublesome and avoidable complications such as bedsores.

When the cause of the paraplegia has been trauma involving the pelvis then a radiological and clinical assessment of the pelvis is obligatory if a vaginal delivery is contemplated.

How would you manage this patient?

I would immediately negotiate with the team from the spinal unit already supervising her care, planning for their involvement should hospital admission become necessary, as well as determining her current status and identifying any current problems.

She is a high risk pregnancy and should be booked for hospital care. Arrangements should be made to facilitate her travel to and from the hospital. I would like to see her weekly throughout pregnancy. Because of the concern regarding the silent onset of labour the cervix should be assessed at each visit from 28 weeks to detect cervical effacement or shortening. She should be admitted at 36 weeks to await the onset of labour unless other obstetric complications demand intervention in their own right. At each visit, a fresh catheter specimen of urine collected by the patient into a suitable sterile container should be submitted for bacteriological culture.

She presents with a urinary tract infection. This could be treated as a single event according to the sensitivities reported; but it would be advantageous to know from those normally responsible for her care and the bacteriologist whether long-term treatment would be indicated. The need for scrupulous perineal toilet and adequate bladder drainage should be emphasized to the patient. If, during the pregnancy, her normal technique prove inadequate then chronic urethral or suprapubic drainage will be required. Good drainage is essential if long-term antibiotics are to be successful. Her renal function as gauged by the creatinine clearance and plasma electrolytes is normal. I would repeat these every 4 weeks or more frequently if they became at all abnormal. Chronic urinary tract infection is associated with refractory iron deficiency anaemia. She should have iron supplements and her haemoglobin and red cell indices checked monthly.

With a flaccid anus and no abdominal tone the patient cannot bear down at stool and therefore it will be necessary to continue with the twice weekly manual evacuation of the bowel by the district team. The stool can be kept soft by a high fibre diet and stool softeners.

The patient gave a well-documented history of deep vein thrombosis and pulmonary embolus treated with anticoagulants. The decision has to be made whether to give the patient prophylactic anticoagulants. Although chairbound it is unusual for paraplegics to develop deep vein thrombosis. The episode was related to her initial injuries and consequent to extensive surgery. It was not related to pregnancy or the oral contraceptive. She is young, in her first pregnancy and not obese. Warfarin crosses the placenta and has been associated with teratogenesis if administered in the first trimester causing chondrodysplasia punctata, and possibly diaphragmatic hernia and the asplenia syndrome. In midpregnancy small intracerebral haemorrhages may cause microcephaly and mental retardation. After 36 weeks retroplacental bleeding may occur and in labour the fetus may suffer severe intracerebral bleeding if the anticoagulation has not been reversed. Long-term heparin administration may result in bone demineralization to which the patient is already prone by virtue of her immobility. Furthermore, heparin prophylaxis has been associated with an increased fetal morbidity. Accordingly I would not prescribe prophylactic anticoagulants. The platelet count is raised presumably as a result of her splenectomy and in the event of immobilization in bed, or the need for caesarean section, subcutaneous heparin should be administered.

Fetal surveillance through pregnancy is as for a normal pregnancy. Repeat ultrasound or cardiotocography being indicated when the clinical picture dictates.

Likewise with the onset of labour, management is dictated by the normal obstetric considerations. Assistance in the second stage may be required because of reduced expulsive efforts owing to the paresis of the abdominal muscles.

Discussion

The level of the spinal defect determines the patient's awareness of labour. With a lesion below T11, T12, or T10 (uterine sensory afferents) the patient will be aware of contractions. From T5 to T10, labour will be painless. Spasticity, flexor spasms or clonus may be aggravated by labour pains. With high lesions above the splanchnic outflow (above T5–T6) there is risk of autonomic hyper-reflexia. An afferent stimulus entering the isolated cord may initiate uninhibited segmental reflexes on a massive scale. Urethral, bladder, rectal and cervical distension, uterine contractions and overbreathing may precipitate this response. Associated acute hypertension mediated by peripheral and splanchnic vasoconstriction may mimic fulminating pre-eclampsia. The patient complains of nasal stuffiness, facial flushing and a pounding headache. Intracranial haemorrhage may occur. The acute hypertension may in turn invoke vagal-mediated bradycardia or arrhythmia. The response to the rapid release of catecholamines is not dissimilar to the paroxysms of phaeochromocytoma. The hypertensive crisis can be controlled by, paradoxically in these patients, spinal or epidural anaesthesia. Amyl nitrate or phentolamine may also be used to control the blood pressure. To avoid such complications developing in labour, patients with high lesions (above T6) are best served by elective caesarean section.

Comment

It is most unlikely that any candidate will have encountered a case such as this in their training but most of the answers required by the examiner could be deduced from background knowledge and experience. The issue of anticoagulation in pregnancy is currently a matter of debate and the candidate would be expected to be aware of the problem and express a personal opinion. It would be easy to panic on receiving such a case but in fact by considering first principles a reasonable plan of management could be described. The phenomenon of autonomic hyper-reflexia is referred to in most of the larger texts but a candidate would not be failed on this alone if unable to answer a question about it. The patient is presented in early pregnancy so that the expected abdominal palpation would not be a major feature of the examination. The candidate might however be asked to demonstrate the essential neurological signs. The emphasis here would be on the taking of a careful and comprehensive history and drawing reasonable conclusions from the data obtained.

Outcome

The patient was admitted to a maternity unit in a hospital with a spinal unit at 36 weeks gestation. Despite the most careful observation, at 37 weeks the onset of labour was heralded by the spontaneous rupture of membranes with the cervix dilated to 7 cm. She progressed rapidly to a normal delivery, the baby weighing 3650 g. There were no third stage complications. The puerperium was uneventful.

Further reading

GREENSPOON, J. S. and PAUL, R. H. (1986) Paraplegia and quadraplegia: special considerations during pregnancy and delivery. *American Journal of Obstetrics and Gynecology*, **155**, 738–741

McGREGOR, J. A. and MEEUWSEN, J. (1985) Autonomic hyper-reflexia: a mortal danger for spinal cord damaged women in labour. *American Journal of Obstetrics and Gynecology*, **151**, 330–333

Case 4

The patient was a 25-year-old bakery worker married for 4 years to her 26-year-old husband, a car mechanic. She was referred to the gynaecology clinic because of menstrual irregularity. She was also a little concerned about an apparent inability to conceive. The couple had used barrier methods for contraception initially, but had been having unprotected intercourse for 12 months. In fact, the couple were not pursuing a pregnancy; the patient's real anxiety was the menstrual irregularity. The husband's work was regular, not taking him from home. There was nothing significant in his medical or surgical history.

The patient's menarche had been at 14 years of age. Until 2 years ago her cycle had been regular, 6–7/26. Since then the cycle had become increasingly irregular varying from 6 weeks to 3 months. She bleeds for between 4 and 7 days. Since starting her job in the bakery 3 years ago, she had put on over 4 stones in weight, which she put down to eating the product between meals! She had noticed that her skin was somewhat greasy but did not complain of hirsutism. There is no history of discharge from the nipples or any visual disturbance. She had no other gynaecological or medical symptoms. There was nothing of significance in her past medical history and she was taking no medication.

On examination her height was 1.51 m and she weighed 66 kg. She was normotensive. She had acne on the face and shoulders. She was not hirsute although the distribution of the pubic hair approached a male escutcheon. The axillary hair was normal and there was no recession of the temple hair line. On confrontation the visual fields appeared intact and there was no neurological deficit demonstrable. There was no goitre and the breasts were normally developed and mature. The abdomen was normal although rather obese, there were no striae. The external genitalia were normal. Pelvic examination confirmed a healthy lower genital tract with a normal cervix. The uterus was of normal size anteverted and mobile. Clinically there were no adnexal masses or tenderness.

Questions

What is your differential diagnosis?

Polycystic ovarian syndrome, hypothyroidism, hyperprolactinaemia, Cushing's syndrome.

The history and examination are suggestive of polycystic ovarian syndrome (PCOS), especially the conjunction of weight gain, infertility and oligomenorrhoea. However both thyroid disease and Cushing's disease can present with a similar picture. Hyperprolactinaemia must always be considered in patients with irregular cycles even if there is no galactorrhoea.

What investigations would you now undertake, and why?

A full blood count	Random blood sugar
Thyroid function tests	Prolactin
Morning plasma cortisol	LH and FSH
Plasma oestradiol	Testosterone and androstenedione
Sex hormone binding globulin (SHBG)	17-hydroxyprogesterone
Ovarian ultrasound	Basal body temperature chart

The thyroid function tests, prolactin and morning plasma cortisol would identify thyroid malfunction, hyperprolactinaemia and Cushing's syndrome. If either the prolactin or morning cortisol were raised then further resting or dynamic tests would be required. An elevated LH concentration and an LH: FSH ratio in excess of 3: 1 would suggest PCOS. The oestradiol level would help to define the method of treatment. Androgens from either the ovary or the adrenal gland can be raised in PCOS and the SHBG can be reduced thus increasing the levels of free testosterone in the blood. The free unbound fraction reflects the increased production of testosterone. The free testosterone fraction may be estimated by dividing the total serum testosterone level by the serum SHBG level and expressing the result as a percentage. This free androgen index normally lies between 0.5% and 19%. Rarely this picture can be mimicked in congenital adrenal hyperplasia of late onset, hence the request for the estimation of the 17-hydroxyprogesterone level which would be raised in this condition. In PCOS ultrasound of the ovaries usually shows a thickened stroma surrounded by a ring of peripheral microcysts of approximately 5–7 mm in diameter. The basal body temperature chart will help to define the cycle length and whether there is an absence of the biphasic pattern suggestive of ovulation.

The following are the results of some of her investigations. What are your conclusions?

TSH:	2.9 mU/l	Androstenedione:	16.2 nmol/l
Thyroxine:	120 nmol/l	SHBG:	25.0 nmol/l
Tri-iodothyronine:	2.0 nmol/l	Prolactin:	283 mU/l
TSH:	4.0 mU/l	Oestradiol:	198 pmol/l
LH:	24.0 U/l	17a-OH-progesterone:	3.8 nmol/l
FSH:	5.3 U/l		
Testosterone:	3.0 nmol/l	Urinary cortisol:	180 nmol/24 h

The patient is euthyroid. The plasma prolactin is normal as is the 24 urinary cortisol and plasma 17-alpha-hydroxyprogesterone.

These results would exclude thyroid disease, hyperprolactinaemia, Cushing's disease and congenital adrenal hyperplasia from the differential diagnosis. The LH to FSH ratio exceeds 3, the level of androstenedione is raised whereas the testosterone level is at the upper level of normal. The sex hormone binding globulin is low but within normal limits. The oestradiol level is within normal limits, the oestrone level which may be raised is not available for comment. The findings are consistent with PCOS.

Yes, and an ultrasound examination confirmed the presence of the characteristic features you described. What advice would you give this patient?

It is still undecided whether weight gain is a primary or a secondary phenomenon in this syndrome. This patient's symptoms were associated with weight gain. However, it is sound advice that she should lose weight and there is evidence that as her height to weight ratio approaches normal she may resume regular ovulation. There is also evidence that treatment will be more effective if she were to lose weight.

What treatment would you recommend?

If she does not wish to conceive it is debateable whether she requires any treatment except to lose weight. If the patient were to request contraceptive advice then a combined oestrogenic oral contraceptive might prevent progression of the condition and it has been claimed that this might make the subsequent induction of ovulation easier. The oral contraceptive has the effect of raising the SHBG level in the blood.

From the point of view of inducing ovulation, anti-oestrogen therapy with clomiphene or tamoxifen remains the first line treatment. This inhibits the negative feedback effects of the elevated unbound oestrogen levels and promotes the production of FSH. Dexamethasone will suppress adrenal hyperandrogenism. If treatment with clomiphene or tamoxifen is unsuccessful then ovulation induction can be attempted by the use of exogenous gonadotrophins. There is a significant risk of ovarian hyperstimulation with the use of exogenous gonadotrophins and pure FSH is less likely to cause ovarian hyperstimulation than human menopausal gonadotrophin. Gonadotrophin releasing hormone analogues (GnRH analogues) by suppressing gonadotrophin secretion may break the dysfunctional pituitary/ovarian cycle allowing a normal endocrine balance to develop.

Discussion

PCOS is a common endocrine disorder. Recent studies show that in women with oligomenorrhoea, using either ultrasound or biochemical criteria, between 80% and 90% have evidence of PCOS. The classical presentation of the Stein–Leventhal syndrome with bilaterally enlarged ovaries, obesity, hirsutism, acne, amenorrhoea/oligomenorrhoea and infertility is rare. The syndrome should be suspected in any woman who presents with oligomenorrhoea, amenorrhoea or hirsutism and who have raised levels of androgens, or an LH:FSH ratio greater than 3:1.

It has been hypothesized that polycystic ovarian syndrome is a self-perpetuating disorder that results from abnormal feedback between the ovary and the hypothalamus and pituitary gland resulting in abnormal gonadotrophin secretion. There is an increase in the pulsatile LH and a relatively low FSH release. Ovarian thecal cells respond with increased androgen production. Normal aromatization of these androgens to 17-beta-oestradiol in the granulosa cells is dependent on FSH. With relative deficiency in FSH there is in the ovary an environment rich in androstenedione and testosterone and reduced 17-beta-oestradiol and this leads to follicular atresia, premature luteinization and anovulation. Circulating sex hormones are reversibly bound to SHBG. If this level is reduced then there will be an increase in the free and active fraction of potent androgens especially testosterone which can promote hirsutism. SHGB levels are reduced in obesity, hypothyroidism and in patients with elevated androgens. The excessive ovarian androgens can be aromatized in peripheral adipose tissue to oestrone. Paradoxically therefore there is a relatively hyperoestrogenic state operating, which with raised androgen exerts both a positive and a negative feedback effect on an essentially normal hypothalamic pituitary axis. The result is the increased LH secretion because of positive feedback and suppressed FSH output because of negative feedback. It has been postulated that these ovaries may also produce increased levels of inhibin which in turn has a specific effect in reducing FSH output further.

These patients are at risk of developing endometrial hyperplasia and in some cases atypical hyperplasia and endometrial adenocarcinoma. Progestogens can be used to promote regular withdrawal bleeds. The preparation should possess low androgenic activity as these patients already have raised levels of androgens. It has been suggested that this train of events might be initiated at the time of puberty as a result of excessive androgen production by the adrenal glands. The aromatase system in adipose tissue converts a proportion of these androgens into oestrone triggering the pituitary response with a high LH, low FSH output to the ovary.

Wedge resection of the ovary was advocated initially because of the mistaken concept that the thickened tunica characteristic of these ovaries might prevent immature follicles ripening and reaching the surface of the ovary. The concept was invalid because such patients can ovulate spontaneously and often respond well to ovulation induction therapy. The operation is invasive and carries with it the risk of adhesion formation which may further compromise the patient's fertility. Ovarian wedge resection still has a place if all medical treatment fails.

Comment

The examination of this patient was absolutely straightforward and consequently the examiners would expect a polished performance in its execution. With a paucity of physical signs their attention will be directed to the evaluation of a differential diagnosis and the management of the condition. With time to spare the questioning might well include an excursion into the biochemical nature of the underlying problem.

Outcome

The patient had not complained at the outset of infertility being a concern for her. During the investigations the couple decided to make the pursuit of pregnancy an immediate priority. Clomiphene was prescribed. On her temperature charts it was established that she commenced ovulation during her second cycle of treatment. Two months later she conceived. The pregnancy was uneventful and breast feeding was established. Following delivery she reverted to her earlier pattern of oligomenorrhoea.

Further reading

ADAM, J., POLSON, D. W. and FRANKS, S. (1986) Prevalence of polycystic ovaries in women with atriovulation and idiopathic hirsutism. *British Medical Journal*, **293**, 355–359

HULL, M. G. R. (1987) Epidemiology of infertility and polycystic ovarian disease: endocrinological and demographic studies. *Gynaecology and Endocrinology*, **1**, 235–245

Case 5

A 26-year-old nurse booked in the antenatal clinic with a history of 21 weeks amenorrhoea. She had a regular menstrual cycle, 5/28. Her last menstrual period had been recorded and she had discontinued the oral contraceptive 6 months before.

She had been delivered of two previous children; the first, a male at term weighing 3450 g and the second, also at term, a female weighing 3460 g. Both pregnancies had been uneventful as were the deliveries although the total duration of the second labour had been only 2 h and 20 min. She was Rhesus negative and had received anti-D gammaglobulin after each delivery.

Her medical history was unremarkable, there was no history of allergy or drug sensitivity. The patient was one of dissimilar twins.

At booking she was well and symptom free. On examination the uterus on palpation was large for dates. Ultrasound confirmed a twin pregnancy appropriate to dates, no congenital abnormalities were identified.

She was booked for hospital antenatal care and arrangements made to see her fortnightly until 27 weeks. The consultant advised admission to hospital at that time until 30 weeks followed by clinic care weekly until the onset of labour. Further ultrasound scans were planned for 28 and 32 weeks.

The patient was unable to make suitable arrangements for the care of her children and therefore did not come into hospital as planned. Antenatal care continued in the clinic.

At 35 weeks the patient referred herself to the hospital. A week before she had wakened in the night with a rigor. Shortly afterwards she vomited. She had felt unwell the day before but had experienced no other symptoms. When seen by her GP her temperature was 37.8°C and routine urinalysis demonstrated one + protein. A provisional diagnosis of urinary tract infection was made and treatment instituted with ampicillin. Culture of the urine was subsequently reported negative. She had come to the hospital because since that episode, although feeling somewhat better she had developed a profound generalized itching which made sleeping difficult. There were no other symptoms although the urine had been a little darker than usual for 48 h. She was unaware of any contact with patients or friends with similar symptoms and in the course of her work had not been exposed to contamination with blood or faecal material. She had not eaten shellfish or taken any drugs.

On examination there was no anaemia or icterus. Her general examination was satisfactory. Abdominal examination suggested that fetal growth had been sustained and this impression was confirmed by ultrasound measurement. Because of the enlarged uterus it was impossible to ascertain whether there was any enlargement of the liver or spleen. There were no changes to be seen in the skin except for some reddening over the shoulders from scratching where the itching had been most intense.

Questions

This patient has developed a generalized pruritis. What is the differential diagnosis?

Jaundice in its various forms especially cholestatic jaundice
Various skin conditions including scabies, pediculosis, urticaria, atopic eczema and neurodermatitis
Drug sensitivities
Hodgkin's disease
Iron deficiency states
Polycythaemia
Carcinoma of the bronchus
Chronic renal failure
Hypothyroidism in association with a dry skin

Look at the following results and bearing in mind the history try to establish a diagnosis.

Hb: 10.3 g/dl, Hct: 0.341,
Red blood cells: 3.69×10^{12}/l,
MCV: 89.1 fl, MCH: 30.1 pg,
MCHC: 33.8 gdl,
White blood cells: 10.3×10^{9}/l.
Hepatitis A specific IgM: not detected
HBs Ag: negative
PT: 14 s, APTT: 41 s, TT: 20 s
Autoimmune antibody screen: negative

Serum electrolytes: normal
Urea: 3.7 mmol/l,
Creatinine: 69 mmol/l,
Total bilirubin: 20 μmol/l,
AST: 276 U/l,
Alk phosphatase: 342 U/l
Albumin: 34 g/l
Abdominal ultrasound: no gall stones seen. Pancreas appears normal.

The only abnormal results are the liver function tests. The alkaline phosphatase is markedly raised even for pregnancy, the total bilirubin is barely elevated and the patient is not icteric. The AST level is 10 times the normal value. The results of the liver function tests do not exclude a viral infection but the history of the condition with the long prodromal pruritus would be unusual. Screening for Hepatitis A and B was negative. There was no history of fatty dyspepsia, there was no tenderness in the epigastrium or gall bladder area and ultrasound has failed to demonstrate any gallstones. An autoimmune hepatitis is unlikely as there were no symptoms in other systems and the autoimmune screen was reported negative. Apart from the rather uncharacteristic increase in liver enzymes the history and laboratory investigations would be consistent with the diagnosis of cholestatic jaundice of pregnancy (intrahepatic cholestasis of pregnancy).

This patient was advised to come into hospital between 27 and 30 weeks. Have you any views on the admission of a patient with a twin pregnancy to hospital in mid pregnancy?

The perinatal mortality of twins is approximately seven times that of singletons. Two major factors are the risk of preterm labour and early intervention because of obstetric complications, notably preeclampsia. On the basis that rest might prevent the development of such complications admission to hospital over the critical period has been advised. Properly controlled studies have not been carried out on a large enough series to prove the assertion although the incidence of preterm labour does seem to relate to the severity and duration of daily work. Preterm labour is associated with social deprivation and it is just this group of patients who cannot come into hospital when required. This patient is not in that category but was unable to make suitable arrangements. In this case the period advised for admission is earlier than usual. Her hospital however is the site of a regional neonatal intensive care unit and this was the period judged to carry the maximal risk to twins in their experience. Whatever the merits of bedrest in preventing the onset of preterm labour or pre-eclampsia, 75% of the perinatal loss occurs before the 33rd week of gestation and therefore it would seem reasonable to have such patients on site when complications develop. For these reasons admission should be offered and the indications discussed with the patient. If the patient were unable to comply with the advice, then weekly assessment of the cervix from 27 weeks, to detect shortening, might help to identify the patient at risk. There is no conclusive evidence that the routine prescription of beta-sympathomimetics or the insertion of a cervical suture earlier in pregnancy improves the prospects for the fetus. The administration of low dose aspirin may prove to be beneficial in preventing the onset of pre-eclampsia.

Discussion

Characteristically intrahepatic cholestasis of pregnancy develops in the last trimester of pregnancy. The presenting symptom is usually increasingly troublesome generalized pruritus. Jaundice may be absent but usually develops 2–4 weeks after the onset of itching. Both jaundice and pruritus subside rapidly after delivery the patient being symptom free within 1–2 weeks. The jaundice is rarely deep, and the stools may be pale and the urine dark. Pain is not usually a feature. Anorexia and malaise may be present.

The serum shows a mild increase in predominantly conjugated bilirubin (total bilirubin usually < 100 μmol/l), with a slight rise in the serum aspartate aminotransferase (AST) and alkaline phosphatase usually within two multiples of the upper limit of normal. In the case described the levels of AST were unusually high. The prothrombin time (PT) may be prolonged because of vitamin K deficiency.

When intrahepatic cholestasis of pregnancy is suspected it is important to first exclude the possibility of viral hepatitis because such cases may present in the cholestatic phase. The serum should be screened for viral markers. Primary biliary cirrhosis is extremely rare in pregnancy. An autoantibody screen would demonstrate mitochondrial antibodies in 95% of such patients and the pruritus would persist after delivery. Ultrasound should be employed to exclude obstruction to the main bile ducts by tumour or gallstones. Liver biopsy is rarely necessary unless the symptoms persist unexpectedly after delivery.

Reports on the prognosis for the baby are conflicting, some series describing an increased incidence of preterm labour, fetal distress and stillbirth. This has been ascribed to bile salts crossing the placenta. Vitamin K deficiency is associated with postpartum haemorrhage. Close monitoring of fetal well being is therefore important.

There is no specific treatment for the condition. Local application of calamine may relieve the pruritus to some extent. If severe, cholestyramine up to 20 g per day may be prescribed. This non-absorbable anion-exchange resin relieves pruritus by binding bile acids and lowering their concentration in the serum. It also binds anionic drugs and vitamin K. Intramuscular vitamin K1 is necessary to control hypoprothrombinaemia.

Distressing though the symptoms may be the timing of the delivery should be dictated by obstetric considerations.

The aetiology of the condition is unknown. It is often familial and studies of pedigree suggest a Mendelian dominant trait. It is likely to recur in subsequent pregnancies and susceptible individuals may develop pruritus on oral contraceptives.

Further reading

FAGAN, E. A. (1989) Intrahepatic cholestasis of pregnancy. In *Medical Disorders in Medical Practice*, 2nd edn, Blackwell Scientific Publications, Oxford, p.433

HALL, M. H. (1990) Rest in hospital and twin pregnancy. *British Journal of Obstetrics and Gynaecology*, **97**, 869–871

McDONALD, A. D., McDONALD, J. C., ARMSTRONG, B., CHERRY, N. M., NOLAN, A. D. and ROBERT, D. (1988) Prematurity and work in pregnancy. *British Journal of Industrial Medicine*, **45**, 56

O'CONNOR, M. C., MURPHY D. and DALRYMPLE, I. K. (1979) Double blind trial of ritodrine and placebo in twin pregnancy. *British Journal of Obstetrics and Gynaecology*, **86**, 707–709

WEEKES, A. R. L., MENZIES, D. N. and DE BOER, C. H. (1977) The relative efficacy of bed rest, cervical suture and no treatment in the management of twin pregnancy. *British Journal of Obstetrics and Gynaecology*, **84**, 161–164

Case 6

The 45-year-old research scientist had been admitted to the medical ward as an emergency. The previous day she had woken up with a cramp-like pain in the right calf. Thinking little of this she had pursued her daily work but noticed progressive swelling of the right calf and foot during the day. Next morning the symptoms were no better and after seeing her GP she was referred to hospital as an emergency with a provisional diagnosis of deep vein thrombosis. She had been symptom free and well until the onset of her symptoms. She did not smoke and had never taken oral contraceptives. She had two children aged 16 and 17 years, both being delivered normally after straightforward pregnancies. Her work was not in any way sedentary and there had been no history of immobilization or trauma to the leg. Her menses were regular, 5/26, although slightly heavy they were not a problem to her and occasioned her only mild discomfort.

Her general examination was that of a normal well-nourished woman apart from the swollen right leg. The swelling involved the whole leg below the knee. The limb was dusky, warm and tender. Peripheral pulses were palpable and there was no loss of sensation or function. A venogram confirmed deep venous thrombosis with obliteration of the femoral vein within the adductor canal and the popliteal and proximal calf veins. A clotting screen and autoimmune screen were reported as normal.

The patient was heparinized. After 48 h, oral anticoagulation was instituted but proved very difficult to stabilize. At this point a pelvic ultrasound was requested to exclude a pelvic cause for the venous thrombosis. The ultrasound examination identified a mass in the right side of the pelvis. Further exploration of the abdomen identified a well-defined echogenic mass 4 cm in diameter in the upper part of the right lobe of the liver in contact with the diaphragm. There was no ascites. A chest X-ray was normal.

On pelvic examination by the gynaecologist the uterus was found to be bulky, anteverted, and displaced forward by a firm mass 10 cm approximately in diameter lying in the pouch of Douglas to the right side. The mass was fixed in the pelvis. On the left side the ovary was enlarged by a cystic swelling 5 cm in diameter. This cyst was mobile. Clinically there was no ascites.

Questions

What is your assessment of the situation to date?

This is a fit symptom-free woman 45 years of age who has presented with a deep vein thrombosis in the right leg. Oral anticoagulation has been difficult to stabilize and she is currently on heparin infusion by pump. There is, on clinical examination bilateral ovarian enlargement with one mass fixed in the pelvis on the same side as the venous occlusion, suggesting that there might be infiltration and involvement of the external iliac vein. An ultrasound examination shows a lesion in the liver.

What is your diagnosis?

Ovarian malignancy with liver metastasis. The liver involvement would indicate Stage IV disease.

When a patient presents with an ovarian tumour, what clinical features would lead you to suspect malignancy?

A history suggesting rapid growth or pain. The likelihood of malignancy is related to the patient's age. Only 20% of tumours discovered before the menopause are malignant. Following that event the risk of malignancy rises to 50–60%. There is loss of weight or failing appetite and in elderly women symptoms of persistent indigestion or dyspepsia. On clinical examination malignancy is suspected if the tumour is solid, or bilateral in distribution. Nodularity in the pouch of Douglas, fixation of the mass suggesting the infiltration of surrounding structures by tumour and ascites are further adverse signs. Unexplained deep vein thrombosis, oedema or varices of the legs or vulva suggesting impaired venous return are other indicators of malignant disease.

Are you therefore certain that this pelvic tumour is malignant?

No. There are some features in this case which do not quite fit. It is unusual for the liver to be a site of parenchymal metastasis in ovarian cancer. Spread is usually to the para-aortic glands, omentum and peritoneum. The supraclavicular node and umbilicus may be involved. If there has been metastatic spread it is unusual for there to be no ascites. The patient has been very well with no suggestion of constitutional upset. In any case, faced with an ovarian mass its nature can never be assumed and a diagnosis should be established by either laparotomy or for persistent small neoplasms, laparoscopy.

Are you advocating laparotomy in this patient at this time?

Laparotomy is essential as soon as it is safe to undertake the procedure. At present her main risk is of pulmonary embolus from an extensive deep vein thrombosis. Continued anticoagulation may cause some resolution of the thrombus and over time the risk of embolus will reduce as the thrombus organizes and what remains becomes more adherent to the vein. It would be helpful to repeat her venogram to confirm resolution of the thrombus to some degree. It would then be possible to plan her laparotomy after switching her anticoagulation to subcutaneous heparin. This small delay is unlikely to worsen her prognosis from the point of view of the ovarian mass. It would also allow further investigations to clarify the situation within the abdomen. More sophisticated imaging with CT scanning or NMR would be helpful to determine the clinical extent of the disease and also to determine the course or possible involvement of the ureters. If these facilities are not available then an IVU would exclude ureteric involvement.

This is the result of a CT scan of the abdomen

The study was taken during an intravenous bolus of 150 ml Niopam®. Two delayed images were obtained of the upper part of the liver 1 h after the bolus.

The pelvic mass consists of a lobulated smoothly encapsulated, apparently solid, mass. The main mass is 10 cm in diameter in the right parametrial region, possibly in the pouch of Douglas and displacing the uterus to the left and compressing the right external iliac veins. There is a smaller 5 cm mass anterior and to the left of the main mass. The rim of these masses shows contrast enhancement. The appearance would fit with ovarian cysts were it not for the ultrasound appearance suggesting a solid mass and the relatively high attenuation (30 HU) on CT scan. There is no evidence of invasion of surrounding tissues.

The previously identified echogenic mass in the liver is seen on the precontrast and immediate postcontrast films. On the delayed postcontrast image, this mass has disappeared indicating vascular filling of the lesion. The findings suggest a solitary cavernous haemangioma of the liver. There is nothing to suggest metastatic disease. The KUB shows an intact urinary tract on both sides.

Do you wish to alter your approach to the case in view of these findings?

No, the CT scan has possibly excluded liver metastasis but her subsequent management depends on the tissue diagnosis of the tumours and an accurate staging at surgery. The apparent absence of infiltration into adjacent tissues by the masses and the absence of ascites is reassuring but the true nature of these masses will only be apparent at laparotomy. The patient requires a total hysterectomy, bilateral salpingo-oophorectomy and omentectomy. All sites involved with residual tumour must be carefully documented. The purpose of the primary operation is to remove all recognizable tumour so as to improve the efficacy of subsequent radiotherapy or chemotherapy.

Discussion

There are a few circumstances where the surgeon has some reluctance in resorting to laparotomy for the evaluation of a persistent ovarian cyst. It is usually taught that a cystic tumour <5–6 cm in diameter can be treated conservatively initially, but explored if it persists for more than 3 months. Most of these in young women are entirely benign and laparotomy would seem excessive. Likewise, in pregnancy most cysts discovered at routine ultrasound are benign. Treatment is desirable to avoid complications such as torsion, haemorrhage or rupture. In pregnancy there are the additional concerns of malpresentation and obstructed labour. It has been advocated that fine needle aspiration under ultrasound control might in such cases be employed to treat such cysts and cytopathological techniques be employed on the aspirate to confirm the diagnosis. The technique is well tolerated and complications are rare.

However, the success of the technique rests on two factors. Initially an ultrasound facility that can identify those features of an ovarian cyst that would suggest neoplasia, and the fact that 100% accuracy is an unrealistic expectation for cytological diagnosis. Compounding two variables is not in the main a sound basis for medical practice but inevitably there have emerged two camps, one of which considers that conservative management is possible after careful selection and the other that this is not sufficiently reliable.

The decision to aspirate will depend at the outset on ultrasonography. To some extent it is assumed that unilocular cysts will be benign, although this may not necessarily be the case. Multilocularity, thick septa and solid areas indicate possible malignancy. False positive rates of 4–27% have been quoted for ultrasound on these criteria, but if the null position is to explore the abdomen in any case this may be considered acceptable. Of greater concern however is the stated false negative rate of up to 9%. False negative reports could lead to inappropriate delay in treatment. In theory these could be identified by positive cytology on aspiration. Malignant cyst fluid usually contains large numbers of malignant cells but the fluid may contain insufficient cells for accurate diagnosis. Necrosis or inflammatory changes and haemorrhage can further obscure the picture. In the group of women under consideration the aim is to identify cysts of follicular origin. Such aspirates should contain normal or luteinized granulosa cells and the fluid should be rich in oestrogen (>4 nmol/l). The identification of epithelial cells indicates the need for removal.

In a small group of patients therefore there would seem to be a place for conservative treatment (aspiration) when small unilocular ovarian cysts (<10 cm diameter) persist in young women or present in early pregnancy. However, the technique must only be employed with a thorough understanding of the limitations of the ultrasound and cytopathological facilities available to the operator. It is imperative that investigations of this kind take place in direct collaboration with the cytopathologist concerned.

In 1988 FIGO revised the staging of ovarian cancer:.

Stage I: Growth limited to the ovaries
- Ia Growth limited to one ovary; capsule intact; no tumour on outer surface; no ascites containing malignant cells.
- Ib Growth limited to both ovaries; capsules intact; no tumour on outer surface; no ascites containing malignant cells.
- Ic Tumour either Ia or Ib, but with tumour on the outer surface, ruptured capsule, or with ascites containing malignant cells or positive peritoneal washings.

Stage II: Growth involving one or both ovaries with pelvic extension
- IIa Extension and/or metastasis to the uterus and/or tubes.
- IIb Extension to other pelvic tissues.
- IIc Tumour either Stage IIa or IIb but with tumour on the surface of one or both ovaries or with capsule(s) ruptured; or with ascites containing malignant cells or with positive peritoneal washings.

Stage III: Tumour involving one or both ovaries with peritoneal implants outside the pelvis and/or positive retroperitoneal or inguinal nodes
- IIIa Tumour grossly limited to the true pelvis with negative nodes but with histologically confirmed microscopic seedings of abdominal peritoneal surfaces.
- IIIb Tumour involves one or both ovaries with confirmed implants of abdominal peritoneal surfaces none exceeding 2 cm diameter. Nodes are negative.
- IIIc Abdominal implants exceed 2 cm in diameter and/or positive retroperitoneal or inguinal nodes.

Stage IV: Growth involving one or both ovaries with distant metastasis

Pleural effusions if present must contain malignant cells and *PARENCHYMAL* liver metastasis falls into this group. *SUPERFICIAL* liver metastasis is classified as Stage III.

Outcome

Following the CT scan the patient remained on intravenous heparin for 12 days during which Doppler examination suggested improvement in the venous return. A repeat venogram confirmed clearance of the femoral vein. There was still some occlusion of the popliteal vein but Doppler confirmed flow around its periphery.

Forty-eight hours before surgery her anticoagulation was changed to s.c. heparin (15 000 units twice daily) reducing to 5 000 units 12 h before her operation.

At operation it was discovered that the right ovary was replaced by a large chocolate cyst 12 cm in diameter. This was adherent to the peritoneum of the pouch of Douglas, the broad ligament on the right and the lateral pelvic wall on that side. The left ovary was likewise replaced by a chocolate cyst 5 cm in diameter. The anatomy was restored by a combination of sharp and blunt dissection and a total hysterectomy and bilateral salpingo-oophorectomy performed.

The pathologist reported that both ovaries were largely replaced by unilocular endometriotic cysts. There was no evidence of malignancy.

The patient's recovery was complete. Hormone replacement therapy was instituted with oestradiol-TTS patches. She was maintained on oral anticoagulants for a further 3 months.

Comment

This is a salutary case because it does demonstrate some of the limitations of even the most sophisticated imaging techniques. These procedures must be interpreted in the context of the complete clinical picture. In the examination the candidate may have to choose between his own clinical diagnosis and that suggested by reports offered by the examiner. The examiner will not try to lead the candidate astray and if a report suggests an alternative diagnosis the candidate should respond by re-examining his own case and covering the arguments for and against the alternative offered. However, in this case the presentation was overwhelmingly in favour of the diagnosis being malignant ovarian disease. The examiner certainly questioned the candidate with this in mind. Endometriosis remains an enigma because its clinical presentation is so unpredictable. This patient manifest none of the usual symptoms associated with that condition despite the presence of massive disease. Conversely, minimal macroscopic disease can produce in some patients profound and incapacitating symptoms.

Further reading

de CRESPIGNY, L. Ch., ROBINSON, H. P., DAVOREN, R. A. M. and FORTUNE, D. (1989) The 'simple' ovarian cyst: aspirate or operate? *British Journal of Obstetrics and Gynaecology*, **96**, 1035–1039

SHEPHERD, J. H. (1989) Revised FIGO staging for gynaecological cancer. *British Journal of Obstetrics and Gynaecology*, **96**, 889–892 (Commentary)

Case 7

This 20-year-old patient was referred to the antenatal clinic by a GP working in a socially deprived area of the city. The family were well known to the support services. Neither she nor her partner had ever been employed; they lived with their two children in a council house. She failed to attend for her first two appointments and the GP was alerted. She eventually attended accompanied by her health visitor at 16 weeks gestation as defined from the date of the last recorded menstrual period. Initially her response to the pregnancy had been to request termination but she then changed her mind. This indecision had caused the delay in her attending the clinic.

She suffered from basilar migraine and had been advised not to take the contraceptive pill. In any case, when taking the oral contraceptive she frequently forgot to take the tablet on time. After the birth of the last child an abnormal cervical smear had been identified. Moderate dysplasia CIN II had been diagnosed on colposcopic biopsy and the lesion treated with CO_2 laser. She had considered a coil for contraception but was unsure as to its suitability after treatment and had not enquired further. She had also defaulted from follow-up in the colposcopy clinic, the cost of travelling to the hospital on public transport being for her a significant item. She was aware that such costs could be reimbursed but felt that the procedure involved too much 'aggravation'. She did not smoke or drink alcohol.

Her first pregnancy 3 years before had caused concern when she failed to gain weight after 33 weeks. She was eventually delivered at term after a normal labour, of a male infant weighing 3800 g. A year later after an uneventful pregnancy she had another normal male baby which weighed 4115 g following a labour of only 3 h at term. Her total weight gain in this pregnancy was 17 kg.

She was 163 cm tall and weighed 55.4 kg. The uterine fundus was palpable above the symphysis pubis consistent with a 15-week gestation. Her haemoglobin was 12.7 g/dl with normal red cell indices.

Two weeks later she remained well. An ultrasound examination reported a single fetus with a BPD of 41 mm and a femur length of 26 mm. No fetal abnormalities were noted and the liquor volume was considered normal for gestation.

The patient was returned to the care of her GP with arrangements to be reviewed again at the hospital at 36 weeks gestation.

At 18 weeks a colposcopic examination of the cervix was normal and she was asked to return for further review after delivery.

On return from shared care, the record showed consistent increase in uterine size throughout the interim. Between 17 and 36 weeks her weight had increased by 9 kg. No problems had occurred. On examination the uterus felt slightly small for dates. The fetus presented by the breech but there appeared to be ample amniotic fluid present. The patient defaulted from her next appointment. The community midwife was notified and she brought the patient back to the clinic at 38 weeks.

There had been no weight gain for 2 weeks. The fundal height was 33 cm. The fetus occupied an oblique lie with the head in the right upper quadrant and the breech high in the left iliac fossa. The back was lowermost. At the time of examination her bladder was empty and she was not constipated. She was admitted to hospital.

Questions

List this patients problems.

The patient's problems are:

Unstable /oblique lie at 38 weeks gestation.
Possible intrauterine growth retardation.
History of rapid delivery.
Contraceptive difficulties.
Poor socioeconomic circumstances.
Need to complete follow-up of treatment for cervical intraepithelial neoplasia.

How would you investigate and manage these problems?

The patient has been admitted at short notice from the antenatal clinic. Because of the difficulties at home the medical social worker and practice health visitor should be notified of the admission, both to mobilize support for the family and to facilitate their access to the hospital. The latter is particularly important to support the mother and alleviate her inevitable anxieties concerning the family's care.

At this gestation, labour or rupture of the membranes may supervene at any time. If the lie is uncorrected then there is the risk of cord prolapse, prolapse of an arm or impaction of the fetus. If neglected, this can lead to uterine rupture or cord compression with fetal death. This patient progressed very rapidly in her last labour and resort to caesarean section may have to be swift. The patient should have blood cross-matched and maintained. The patient and the ward staff must be instructed to summon help immediately should rupture of the membranes be suspected.

The cause of the oblique lie should be identified. Her initial ultrasound report failed to identify the location of the placenta. *Placenta praevia* must be excluded by pelvic ultrasound. The same examination should eliminate the possibility of *major fetal abnormality, acquired pelvic pathology* (such as ovarian cyst), *fibroids* or *excess amniotic fluid.* The patient's two previous recent pregnancies had been normal and therefore a *uterine anomaly* or a significantly *contracted pelvis* are unlikely, the latter especially, as her last baby weighed 4115 g and was delivered normally after a short labour.

The failure to gain weight and the discrepancy in fundal height might suggest intrauterine growth retardation (IUGR). In such a case the unstable lie could result solely from there being a small baby in a uterus stretched by the previous pregnancy. Having excluded placenta praevia, then a pelvic examination could identify pelvic contraction but in this case it would be academic.

The uterus grows in three dimensions during pregnancy and therefore too much emphasis can be placed on measurements in one dimension, e.g. symphysial fundal height, especially when the lie of the fetus is other than longitudinal. A more precise estimate of fetal weight can be made after measurement by ultrasound of the fetal head circumference and abdominal circumference. A diminished liquor pool would also suggest IUGR. If growth retardation is suggested by such measurements then delivery is indicated. If fetal cardiotocography is normal then a vaginal delivery could be attempted after a stabilizing induction. If abnormal, then delivery by caesarean section would be indicated.

If IUGR is reasonably excluded then a conservative management can be instituted. As a precaution, serial fetal cardiotocography will reassure the patient and her attendants as to the current well-being of the fetus. The expectancy is that as term approaches, the increasing tone in the uterus will stabilize the lie of the fetus longitudinally. If this happens before the onset of labour the patient can be allowed home. However, she has a history of rapid labour, and a case can be made to keep her in hospital to await the onset of labour for fear of delivery in inappropriate circumstances.

External cephalic version during the unstable phase is unlikely to result in any lasting advantage and could be prejudicial to the fetus. Once the lie has stabilized at this gestation then induction of labour by rupture of the membranes would be in order. Should the patient go past term with the lie still unstable then a decision would have to be made to undertake a stabilizing induction of labour. The timing depends on a number of factors, not least, the patient's probable increasing anxiety as she has to tolerate a situation that she understands to be hazardous to her baby. Eventually the indication of postmaturity itself becomes relevant. With the passage of time and failure of the lie to stabilize spontaneously, the risk of the membranes rupturing and the cord or a limb prolapsing increases. The decision made, external cephalic version is performed to correct the lie. Syntocinon is given intravenously starting with very low concentrations in order to improve uterine tone and promote contractions. Caution is required because of the risk of a dramatic response in a sensitive patient resulting in tonic contraction and uterine rupture, especially if the lie once again becomes abnormal. When the head is considered to be stabilized in the pelvic brim then low amniotomy can be performed, preferably in theatre, in case the cord prolapses and emergency caesarean section is required. The release of liquor should be as controlled as possible.

How would you tackle this patient's difficulty with contraception? Would you advise tubal ligation in the event of a caesarean section being performed?

This pregnancy was unplanned and initially the patient's response was to seek a termination . A further pregnancy in her current situation would be a disaster. Ideally her intentions for future contraception should have been established early in pregnancy to avoid her having to make vital decisions later, under pressure, when complications develop. I do not think that this is the time to propose tubal ligation. She is only 20 years old and the family is socially and financially stressed. In this situation marital breakdown is common. The outcome of this pregnancy is as yet uncertain. The efficacy of tubal ligation is reduced if performed at caesarean section rather than as an interval procedure. Likewise, reversal of sterilization is less likely to be successful, should she subsequently request it, if the operation were undertaken at caesarean section or in the immediate puerperium. At an interval procedure, laparoscopy with the application of clips or rings, is associated with less tissue damage thus facilitating a more successful reversal. In a woman of this age, despite her pressing problems, this is an essential consideration. Consequently, although aware of her difficulties with contraception I would not *advise* tubal ligation should a caesarean section be necessary. Should this patient request a tubal ligation before intervention then these points must be discussed. Assuming that tubal ligation is not performed at delivery then some plan for contraception must be initiated before the patient leaves hospital. An oral contraceptive would be unsuitable because of the patient's admitted unreliability in taking her tablets. An IUCD could be fitted at a postnatal examination. This would be best arranged with her GP or local clinic as her attendance at hospital tends to be unpredictable. Sheaths would not be reliable enough for this patient.

My preference would be to meet with the patient and her husband 3 months after delivery to explore all options with them including tubal ligation and vasectomy. During the interim I would prescribe depot progesterone for her. The views of her GP, health visitor, and social worker could be solicited, so that in the event of a sterilization being agreed to in such a young woman, all her circumstances would have been properly considered.

Comment

There is nothing complicated in this case. The problems listed are those that any obstetrician meets every day in clinical practice. The question on tubal ligation was designed to explore the candidates attitudes and sensitivity to a particular patient's needs. The examiner might not personally agree with the response but it would be perfectly acceptable for the reasons given. It would have been an error to say no to the question without being prepared to explain why. This description has not explored all the possibilities for discussion in this case and it would be a useful exercise for a potential candidate to consider what other avenues of questioning might be derived from this history.

Outcome

At term plus 2 days the fetus was presenting by the head over the pelvic brim. There appeared to be some increased tone in the uterus. A Syntocinon infusion was commenced and when contractions started an amniotomy was performed in theatre with a controlled release of amniotic fluid. The fluid was clear. The patient was returned to the labour ward where, despite the

Syntocinon infusion contractions remained desultory. Four hours later when re-examined the lie was again oblique with the head in the right iliac fossa. A caesarean section was performed with the delivery of a baby weighing 2780 g, significantly less than her previous baby.

Case 8

The 80-year-old patient had complained of vulval irritation for 3 or 4 years. The symptom had become noticeably worse 2 months before she appeared in the out-patient department. The itch had become very intense and to her embarrassment caused her to scratch the vulval area in order to gain a measure of relief, especially at night. There had been no bleeding and no discharge per vaginum or per rectum. She had used a number of applications to relieve her symptoms including TCP ointment, zinc and castor oil cream and calamine lotion. None of these had either relieved or exacerbated her symptom. She was a widow, a retired headmistress. She lived alone but managed perfectly well and in particular enjoyed a varied and adequate diet. Her menarche had been at the age of 13 years of age, the menstrual cycle during her adult life had been normal, and the menopause had supervened at 50 years of age. She only had only one child, a son, delivered normally after a straightforward pregnancy. No other pregnancies ensued and therefore she decided to pursue her career in teaching. Apart from a road traffic accident 5 years before she had had no cause to consult her doctor. She had no known allergies or sensitivities and was on no known medication.

On examination, she was a well-nourished woman weighing 60 kg. Her height was 150 cm. She was not anaemic and her general examination was satisfactory. The abdomen was normal to palpation with no organomegaly.

On inspecting the vulva it was seen to be atrophic. The tissues were not swollen and there were no scratch marks. In the midline just above the clitoris there was a slightly raised lesion 2 cm in the longitudinal axis × 1 cm. The lesion was red in colour with some white hyperkeratotic patches. It was not fixed and moved freely over the deeper tissues. It appeared to be limited to the epidermis. There was no bleeding from the site and the tissues did not appear to be indurated. There was no inguinal lymphadenopathy. A speculum examination confirmed an atrophic vagina, the cervix was normal and a bimanual examination demonstrated no abnormalities.

Questions

Can you identify the nature of this vulval lesion, have you seen anything like it before?

No, the nature of the lesion is not apparent from its appearance.

How do you intend to proceed?

Because the nature of the lesion is uncertain excision biopsy is necessary to exclude malignant change.

What malignant lesions may be encountered on the vulva?

The most common is squamous cell carcinoma. Basal cell carcinoma is much rarer. These lesions tend to present in the menopausal patient. Melanomas can present in the younger woman as can sarcomas. The vulva can also be the site of metastatic growth usually blood borne. Carcinoma of the breast may present in this way or recurrence manifest itself often long after the primary treatment. Very rarely the vulva may be involved with non-Hodgkin's lymphoma or leukaemia. In addition carcinoma of Bartholin's gland is a rare possibility.

How do primary lesions of the vulva spread?

The squamous cell carcinoma spreads by local extension to involve the vagina, urethra and anus. Lymphatic dissemination is first to the superficial inguinal nodes. From here further spread can occur to the deep inguinal (femoral), pelvic external iliac, and obturator nodes. It has been suggested in the past that involvement of the clitoris by tumour made spread to the pelvic lymphatics more likely. This has not been confirmed. Involvement of the pelvic (deep) lymph glands appears to be related to the size of the vulval carcinoma. Lesions > 4 cm in any diameter are most likely to have pelvic node metastasis. Unilateral tumours usually metastasize to the inguinal glands on both sides.

Basal cell tumours extend by local infiltration and in the main this process is slow. It does not metastasize.

Melanomas metastasize to the groin nodes in the same way as the squamous carcinomas but the timing of this phenomenon is very variable. The spread can be extremely rapid or the lesion may lie dormant for many years.

Sarcomas metastasize via the blood stream and involvement of the lymph glands is unusual.

What are the principles that dictate the surgical management of malignant disease of the vulva?

The surgery is defined by an understanding of the mode of spread of the lesion concerned. For squamous cell carcinoma the basic operation should be a radical vulvectomy and bilateral groin node dissection. Palpation of the nodes is a poor index of their actual involvement so that failure to palpate glands does not imply a limitation of the procedure. The morbidity of the operation is increased once the dissection is extended upwards retroperitoneally after dividing the inguinal ligaments to retrieve the deep inguinal glands. As there is no evidence that these glands are involved without first involving the groin nodes the deep dissection should be reserved for lesions $\geqslant$ 4 cm in diameter. A number of techniques have been employed to try and identify involved pelvic glands before surgery. Ultrasound, computed tomography, magnetic resonance imaging, lymphangiography and image guided fine needle aspiration have been attempted but with no reliable results upon which to base management. Because the radical operation is mutilating there has been some debate as to whether small Stage I lesions placed laterally and not impinging on midline structures can be treated by vulvectomy and ipsilateral groin dissection. The situation is unclear and until the case is proven bilateral groin dissection remains the preferred option.

For basal cell carcinoma simple vulvectomy should suffice. Melanomas demand vulvectomy and bilateral groin dissection and the rare sarcoma is dealt with by vulvectomy alone. Malignant change in Bartholin's gland requires radical vulvectomy with block dissection of the inguinal glands on both sides.

Do you know how successful surgery can be in the treatment of squamous cell carcinoma of the vulva?

The success depends on the node involvement. Figures have been quoted as high as 72% survival rate overall at 5 years. If the inguinal nodes are negative the 5-year survival rate rises to 94% but falls to 62% if they are involved. Involvement of the pelvic nodes dramatically reduces the prognosis the 5-year survival being in the order of only 20%.

Does radiotherapy have a place in the treatment of vulvar carcinoma?

Very little. The vulval tissues are very sensitive to ionizing radiation so that a cancerocidal dose produces a violent and persistent reaction in the surrounding skin. Its use is therefore limited to the palliative treatment of patients considered to be inoperable, to reduce tumour bulk before surgery, especially when adjacent structures such as the rectum are involved, and as an adjunct to surgery when pelvic nodes are involved and complete removal may be uncertain.

This lady complained of pruritis vulvae. Apart from your obvious concern about the lesion discovered on the vulva, would you undertake any other investigations?

There is no certainty that the lesion is responsible for her symptoms. *Trichomonas* and *Candida* infections should be excluded by the taking of high vaginal swabs. Elderly patients may develop a bacterial vaginal discharge in association with senile vaginitis. This usually causes pain and soreness rather than itch. This patient is very specific as to the nature of her discomfort and scratching was a feature of her history. Vulval itching can be the dominant symptom in a more generalized pruritis. A full blood count, urea and electrolytes, and serum bilirubin levels should exclude pruritis resulting from lymphoma, jaundice or uraemia. Anaemia with abnormalities in the red cell indices may draw attention to deficiency states which can cause pruritis. Vitamin B12, folate and iron deficiency can all be a cause. If present, further tests for malabsorption are indicated including the identification of achlorhydria. Atopy from local allergies to soaps, bath salts, deodorants, washing powders, lotions or fabrics can be identified by a careful history directed at detecting changes in her habits that coincided with the onset of symptoms. If suggested, then skin sensitivity tests can confirm the diagnosis. Hyperglycaemia with or without glycosuria can be responsible for the symptom and glycosuria because of reduced renal threshold can do the same. Ideally a glucose tolerance test should be performed. Skin disease not specific to the vulva may be responsible. Although the vulva may be extensively involved a careful search should be made of other sites for psoriasis, scabies or seborrhoeic dermatitis. The chronic vulval dystrophies are associated with severe often protracted and intractable pruritis. Diagnosis is by tissue biopsy.

What do you mean by chronic vulval dystrophy?

The skin of the vulva is commonly the site of chronic changes the aetiology of which is obscure. In the past depending on the colour of the abnormal area, its distribution, and its thickness it was diagnosed as leucoplakia, lichen sclerosis or kraurosis. Unfortunately these lesions did not correlate with specific histological criteria and indeed in any given case different histological patterns might be apparent. Three histological variants emerge:

1. Hyperplastic dystrophy: with hyperkeratosis at the surface and a thicker acanthotic epithelium. There is an associated chronic inflammatory cell infiltrate.
2. Lichen sclerosis (atrophic dystrophy): there is epithelial atrophy. Hyperkeratosis is present but below the epithelium is usually a homogenous featureless layer. A chronic inflammatory cell infiltrate is also present.
3. Mixed dystrophy: a combination of the features of both the previous pictures with acanthosis and a subepithelial homogenous zone and/or it has been suggested adjacent areas of these two types.

Nuclear atypia can develop in any of these variants leading to the varieties of vulval epithelial neoplasia and carcinoma *in situ*.

How do you treat pruritis caused by vulval dystrophy?

Symptomatic relief is only indicated when premalignant or malignant change has been excluded. The risk of carcinoma developing from vulval dystrophy is 1–5%. Such change is always preceded by the development of atypia within the epithelium. Consequently, providing that the initial biopsies show no dysplasia, treatment can be directed to symptomatic relief. Whatever treatment is applied all patients require continuous supervision for life. The clinical features should be carefully documented and changes assessed by biopsy. Once all possible contributory causes for pruritis have been excluded or treated in their own right then the initial treatment of the dystrophy should be medical. Hyperplastic dystrophies respond well to hydrocortisone cream (0.5%). Testosterone ointment has been suggested for atrophic lesions but note must be taken of clitoral enlargement and facial hirsuties. A surge in libido can be embarrassing for the patient. Oral hydrochloric acid may produce a subjective response even if achlorhydria has been excluded. Simple vulvectomy remains only for the most intractable cases. The disease is multifocal and often recurs beyond the limits of the original excision. Vulvectomy, skinning vulvectomy, and laser therapy are best reserved for those cases where vulval epithelial neoplasia is shown to be present or which develops subsequently.

Discussion

There has been a revision of the FIGO staging for vulval cancer. It is based upon the TNM non-operative method of staging:

T *Relates to the primary tumour.*
Tis Preinvasive carcinoma, carcinoma *in situ.*
T1 Tumour confined to the vulva and/or perineum, <2 cm in maximum dimension.
T2 Tumour confined to the vulva and/or perineum, >2 cm in maximum dimension.
T3 Tumour of any size with adjacent spread to urethra and/or vagina and/or anus.
T4 Tumour of any size infiltrating bladder mucosa and/or rectal mucosa including the upper urethral mucosa and/or fixed to bone.
N *Relates to the regional lymph nodes.*
N0 No nodes palpable.
N1 Unilateral inguinal lymph node metastasis.
N2 Bilateral inguinal lymph node metastasis.
M *Relates to distant metastasis.*
M0 No clinical metastasis.
M1 Distant metastasis including pelvic lymph node metastasis.

Using this format the staging advised is as follows:

Stage 0:	Tis	Carcinoma *in situ*, intraepithelial carcinoma
Stage I:	T1 N0 M0	
Stage II:	T2 N0 M0	
Stage III:	T3 N0 M0	Tumour of any size with adjacent
	T3 N1 M0	spread to the lower urethra and/
	T1 N1 M0	or vagina, or the anus, and/or unilateral regional lymph node
	T2 N1 M0	involvement

Stage IVA:	T1 N2 M0 T2 N2 M0	Tumour invades any of the following: upper urethra, bladder mucosa, rectal mucosa, pelvic bone
	T3 N2 M0	and/or bilateral regional lymph node involvement
	T4 N1/N2 M0	
Stage IVB:	Any T, Any N, M1	Any distant metastasis including pelvic lymph nodes

There are certain limitations in the application of this classification when one considers the factors listed above that dictate the surgical procedures. The size of tumour designated for staging is only 2 cm in the maximum dimension. Results show that the pelvic glands need only be removed when the lesion is larger than this, i.e. > 4 cm. The staging is dependent on the palpation of lymph nodes. This is notoriously inaccurate as a measure of lymph node involvement. In one series of 208 patients with vulval carcinoma the inguinal glands were impalpable in 153; in 35 of these (23%) the glands were histologically positive. Likewise, in the same series, in 54 cases the nodes were palpable and in 30 (55%) the nodes were histologically free of growth. No account is made of the location of the tumour, and it has been suggested that laterally situated tumours of small size might be treated by vulvectomy and ipsilateral node resection. Finally, no account has been taken of the histology of the tumour. Some growths, e.g. melanomas may be < 2 cm diameter but may still be extremely aggressive and carry a poor prognosis. A surgical/histological staging has been implemented for corpus carcinoma because of the improved prognostic indication that results. The same consideration would seem necessary for vulval carcinoma.

Outcome

An excision biopsy of the localized lesion was taken. The histological report confirmed a superficial basal cell carcinoma. A simple vulvectomy was performed, no residual basal cell carcinoma was seen in the operation specimen. The vulval skin was normal with no atypia. Following removal of the lesion her pruritis resolved. Four years later she presented with a procidentia and a vaginal hysterectomy was undertaken. She was still free of any vulval symptoms and on examination the residual vulval skin was normal.

Comment

Cases presented to candidates need not be in any way 'difficult'. The history here was simple, the findings obvious and straightforward. The examiner clearly then is going to stress in the viva component the actual management of the case and explore possible areas of controversy. Candidates are frequently unsure about the concept of the chronic vulval dystrophies. The essential fact is that diagnosis can only be established by tissue biopsy and that it is somewhat futile to attempt to allocate the patient to one or other of the now obsolete clinical entities. Unfortunately the histological classification of the vulval dystrophies remains a subject of discussion and nomenclature may change. The concept of a hypertrophic and a hypotrophic group of dystrophies is likely to persist although the exact names for these categories may be amended. The management of pruritis remains largely empirical once associated causes have been excluded. It is reasonable for the examiner to expect the candidate to know a few basic statistics about survival of patients at the different stages of malignant disease.

Further reading

JEFFCOATE, T. N. A. and WOODCOCK, A. S. (1961) Premalignant lesions of the vulva with particular reference to clinical epithelial dystrophies. *British Medical Journal*, **ii**, 127–134

LAVERY, H. A. (1984) Vulval dystrophies: new approaches. In *Clinics in Obstetrics and Gynaecology*, Vol. 11, No. 1 (ed. H. Fox), W. B. Saunders Company, London, pp. 155–169

MONAGHAN, J. M. (1986) Radical surgery for carcinoma of the vulva. In *Bonney's Gynaecological Surgery* (ed. J. M. Monaghan) 9th edn, Balliere Tindall, London, pp. 121–127

MONAGHAN, J. M. (1987) Vulvar carcinoma: the case for individualisation of treatment. In *Bailliere's Clinical Obstetrics and Gynaecology*, Vol. 1, No. 2, Balliere Tindall, London, pp. 263–276

WAY, S. (1948) The anatomy of the lymphatic drainage of the vulva, and its influence on the radical operation for carcinoma. *Annals of the Royal College of Surgeons of England*, **3**, 187

Case 9

The patient was a 26-year-old Caucasian machine operator married to a dispatch rider. This was her first pregnancy. She attended the antenatal clinic 19 weeks after the last recorded menstrual period. This had been 3 weeks later than expected and was lighter than usual. Apart from this variation her cycle had always been regular, 7/28. She had used the oral contraceptive for a year in all stopping 9 months before the last period. She had not felt fetal movements. Her GP's letter referred to an examination 2 weeks before her appointment when the uterine size was considered to be 'consistent with her dates'.

Her past medical history and family history were unremarkable. She was taking no drugs but smoked 30 cigarettes per day and took alcohol only in small amounts and very infrequently.

On examination she was of small stature, height 152 cm, weight 50.2 kg. Her general examination was otherwise normal, blood pressure 130/70 mmHg. Abdominally, the uterine fundus was palpable at a level compatible with a 16-week pregnancy and this was the impression also on bimanual examination. An ultrasound examination showed a single fetus occupying a transverse lie. The placenta was situated in the fundus. The BPD was 3.5 cm and the femur length 2.2 cm. There were no fetal anomalies.

These measurements were consistent with a gestation of 16 weeks. The EDD was adjusted and the patient returned to the care of her GP until 34 weeks gestation. The investigations were as follows:

Hb:	14.6 g/dl	Rubella:	Immune
Normal indices:		Cervical smear:	Negative
VD serology:	Negative	Urinalysis:	Negative

The patient failed to return to the hospital at 34 weeks as planned. Eventually the community midwife established contact and brought her to the hospital clinic at 36 weeks gestation. She had not attended her GP or local clinic during the interim as she had felt very well. She had not responded to notes left at her address by the practice staff. She was examined in the clinic and told that the baby was smaller than expected and advised to come into hospital for further investigations.

She is now at 37 weeks on dates established by the ultrasound measurements at her first visit. Her weight is 55 kg. She is normotensive, blood pressure 120/80 mmHg. Her urinalysis is normal on dipstick testing. On abdominal examination the uterine fundus is palpable four fingers breadth below the xiphisternum. The fundal/symphysial separation is 31 cm. The fetus occupies a longitudinal lie with the head presenting. The head has not engaged in the pelvis, 3/5 of the head being palpable above the pelvic brim. The fetal parts are clearly felt, there appears to be little liquor present. Fetal movements can be seen and the fetal heart rate is 130 beats/min and regular.

Questions

What is the diagnosis?

Clinically the baby is 'small for dates'. Without more information a precise diagnosis is not possible. Possibilities include:

1. An error in the estimation of gestational age. This is unlikely because although her menstrual history was suspect, an ultrasound examination was performed early in pregnancy at 16 weeks gestation, when estimates of gestational age are at their most reliable.
2. This could be a small baby because of some inherent defect (chromosomal abnormality, renal agenesis, etc.) or insult in early pregnancy during the period of organogeny, e.g. maternal infection by rubella.
3. This picture could indicate intrauterine growth retardation (IUGR) and uteroplacental insufficiency.
4. This could be a small baby in a small patient realizing its genetically determined growth potential.

Apart from severe congenital abnormality, the greatest risk to the baby would be IUGR and the possibility of intrauterine anoxia and intrauterine death.

We have no records to tell us whether the discrepancy between uterine size and gestation is of recent origin. Likewise although her apparent weight gain has been only 5 kg since 16 weeks, there is no record of the pattern of weight change during the interim. IUGR is associated with cigarette consumption and she is a heavy smoker. She has not experienced any of the complications of pregnancy associated with IUGR, e.g. hypertensive and renal disorders, bleeding in early pregnancy or antepartum haemorrhage. Urinalysis is normal and there was no family history of diabetes. She is, however, small herself and is more likely to have a small baby whose weight would be in the lower range of a normal population. Assuming, therefore, that the estimation of gestational age on the early ultrasound is correct, the history and clinical examination cannot distinguish between the high risk (IUGR, fetal abnormality/compromized fetus) and lower risk categories.

How would you have managed the situation as it presented at 36 weeks?

I would admit the patient to hospital explaining that her baby felt smaller than expected and although this might prove to be of no consequence at all, there are conditions which would demand closer observation and possibly an early delivery.

Assuming initially that the problem was IUGR I would request that the patient be rested in bed to promote placental blood flow. She would be advised to stop smoking.

In addition to routine ward observations for fetal well-being I would request that she start recording fetal movements on a Fetal Activity (kick) chart. Fetal cardiotocography would be requested on alternate days. If the facilities were available I would ask for fetal ultrasound with biophysical profile if possible each week. Further investigations would include a TORCH screen, and a random blood sugar.

The ultrasound scan performed at 36 weeks when she was admitted was reported as follows:

BPD: 8.3 cm (+/- 0.1 cm), HC: 29.0 cm, AC: 27.6 cm, Liquor pool maximum depth: 6 cm. Heart, spine, kidneys and bladder visualized and normal.

From the charts provided (see Appendices II and III), for 36 weeks the measurement for the BPD lies below two standard deviations of the mean. This result confirms the clinical impression that the baby is small. The head and abdominal circumferences occupy a similar position when plotted against gestational age. The HC to AC ratio is closer to unity. The liquor pool is adequate. These measurements do not identify asymmetrical growth retardation suggestive of uteroplacental insufficiency. Immediate intervention to deliver the baby is not indicated. This picture of symmetrical growth retardation is nevertheless associated with an increased perinatal mortality. A single measurement does not reveal the dynamics of fetal growth and the investigation should be repeated. Although major fetal abnormalities appear to be absent, the picture is still consistent with a chromosomal anomaly. If severe growth retardation had been evident earlier in pregnancy then amniocentesis would have been appropriate to exclude fetal abnormalities of this kind. At this gestation amniocentesis would not provide an answer in time to influence management. Cordocentesis would provide answers more quickly but carries an increased risk to the fetus. With this relatively small degree of growth impairment on ultrasound measurement the risk is probably not justified. The concern is the risk of delivering an abnormal baby by caesarean section in the event of fetal distress supervening in labour.

Describe your management from this point.

Babies who are preterm as well as growth retarded have the highest perinatal mortality rates. It is an advantage to sustain the pregnancy to 38–39 weeks if possible. The patient should remain in hospital where the fetus can be delivered promptly whatever the gestational age . The frequent assessment of fetal well-being is mandatory. The aim should be to await the onset of spontaneous labour or achieve 38–39 weeks whichever is the sooner. At 38–39 weeks labour should be induced. Intervention is indicated earlier to deliver the baby if there is any suggestion of asymmetrical growth supervening, i.e. increase in the HC to AC ratio, or a falling away from the two standard deviations value. Intervention would also be indicated if there were any adverse features on the fetal ECG trace.

Discussion

The commonest definition of intrauterine growth retardation (IUGR) is 'Birthweight less than the 10th centile for gestational age and sex'. If the data base for this defined population included only normal pregnancies with normal outcomes then clearly 10% of normal pregnancies would be so categorized. If the population included all cases, excluding perhaps twins, then even so the IUGR group would include some normal cases. By defining such a group it is hoped to include those babies in whom growth is truly impaired, i.e. those babies in whom incremental growth with time is less than acceptable. IUGR infants are recognized as having increased perinatal and infant morbidity and mortality, as well as an increased prevalence of developmental and physical growth handicap. A single measurement of *size* is therefore not enough to establish the diagnosis and serial measurements are required to reveal the rate of growth compared with the normal. Babies with birthweights below the 10th centile may be small for gestational age without being growth retarded. The definition employed demands an *accurate* assessment of gestation and would not identify those babies whose weight drops from the 90th centile to the 20th over a short period. Such a fetus could be in immediate peril whereas a fetus sustaining a normal growth rate along the 8th centile would be at less risk. As yet charts plotting incremental changes in fetal parameters have not been universally adopted. The measurement of the abdominal circumference or HC to AC ratio resolves the dilemma in some cases by identifying the end result of uteroplacental insufficiency, i.e. head sparing. To the same end Doppler studies of fetal aortic, or umbilical artery blood flow, and in particular the demonstration of reduced or absence of end diastolic blood flow, serve to identify the small baby with fetoplacental impairment.

The diagnosis of IUGR is missed in 50–75% of cases. The reason is probably the necessity first to recognize clinically that the problem may exist. Clinical sensitivity can be heightened by an appreciation of maternal risk factors. A past history of a previous IUGR baby, perinatal death, congenital abnormality, recurrent abortion, or preterm labour are important indicators of the increased likelihood of IUGR in the current pregnancy. Likewise, maternal factors such as hypertension, renal disease, recurrent urinary tract infection, cardiopulmonary conditions, sickle disease and the development of pre-eclampsia should suggest increased fetal surveillance. Cigarette smoking or abuse of alcohol, methadone or heroin also contribute to the risk. Clearly many complications of pregnancy will put the fetus at risk and demand monitoring of fetal development *in utero* in their own right. Sixty-seven % of IUGR infants are born to mothers exhibiting at least one risk factor in their history .

Abdominal palpation is still used by some to assess fetal growth and size. Repeated studies have shown it to be grossly inaccurate, errors being greatest at the extremes of fetal weight where the information is most needed. Maternal weight gain is taken to reflect fetal growth. Providing that the patient is weighed under controlled conditions at each visit, minimizing between apparatus and between observer variables as well as vagaries of dress, there may be some correlation. In reality, the recording of weight in many clinics is a lottery.

The fundal height measured in centimetres from the upper border of the symphysis to the top of the uterine fundus has been used to record uterine (and therefore fetal) growth in a reproducible and significant manner. Assessments of intra- and interobserver variation differ. In spite of this, measurement of the fundal height has been reported to have a good sensitivity for identifying small birthweight babies for gestation (proportion of small babies detected) and also a satisfactory specificity (proportion of normal weight babies identified as such). Remembering that the identification of a small birthweight baby is not synonymous with the detection of a growth retarded baby the measurement can be usefully employed as a screening test leading to more objective examination by ultrasound.

Ultrasound studies have been directed principally to the measurement of fetal size and the detection of the small baby. A better index of fetal compromise would be the detection of disturbances in fetal growth velocity.

Comment

The situation described is common in clinical practice. The physical signs are easily demonstrated. The danger is to rush to a diagnosis which is not established by the evidence available. To diagnose this case as intrauterine growth retardation at the outset, implying uteroplacental insufficiency, would have been an error. The examiner was interested in the interpretation of episodic ultrasound data and its application to a dynamic and changing situation such as fetal growth.

Outcome

At 38 weeks the ultrasound examination was repeated. BPD: 8.7 cm, HC: 31.7 cm, AC: 30 cm. The maximum liquor pool was 5.8 cm, Active fetal breathing was observed.

Labour was induced at the end of the 39th week. At ARM clear liquor drained. The first stage lasted 9 hours, delay was encountered in the second stage and the baby was delivered by midcavity forceps. The baby weighed 2210 g and had an Apgar score of 8 at 1 minute.

Further reading

BEAZLEY, J. M. and KURJAK, A. (1973) Prediction of foetal maturity and birthweight by abdominal palpation. *Nursing Times*, 14 June, 763–765

CALVERT, J. P., CREAN, E. E., NEWCOMBE, R. G. and PEARSON, J. F. (1982) Antenatal screening by measurement of symphysis-fundus height. *British Medical Journal*, **285**, 846–849

DETER, R. L., HARRIST, R. B., BIRNHOLZ, J. C. and HADLOCK, F. P. (eds) (1986) *Quantitative Obstetrical Ultrasonography*, John Wiley, New York

SHOLL, J. S., WOO, D., RUBIN, J. M., LIN C.-C. and MOAWAD, A. H. Intrauterine growth retardation risk detection for fetuses of unknown gestational age. *American Journal of Obstetrics and Gynecology*, **144**, 709–714

VILLAR, J. and BELIZAN, J. M. (1986) The evaluation of the methods used in the diagnosis of intrauterine growth retardation. *Obstetrical and Gynecological Survey*, **41**, 187–199

Case 10

A 45-year-old shop assistant was referred by her GP to the out-patient department with symptoms of perineal discomfort and a lump 'down below'. She had been well until 3 months before when her husband had a minor stroke and was made bedbound. This involved her nursing him and assisting in moving him from the bed to a chair or commode and back again. She became conscious in the beginning only of a 'fullness' at the introitus but was alarmed to see a swelling emerging from the vagina when she went to the toilet. She experienced a dragging discomfort in the lower abdomen. This became worse as the day progressed and by evening she usually developed sacral backache. This was localized to the lower sacrum and there was no radiation down the legs. She admitted to no urinary symptoms, and had no problems in evacuating her bowels. All her symptoms resolved when finally she laid down in bed at night. During the day they became progressively worse, to the extent that she could no longer cope with her work and the added responsibility of her husband, despite the GP having arranged home nursing during the day for him.

Her menses were regular, 6/21, and slightly heavier of late but not excessive. She had two children, both away at university. Her pregnancies had been normal and her deliveries normal as far as she knew. Their birthweights had been 3500 g and 3900 g. She had used the cap for contraception since the birth of the second child but intercourse had stopped when her husband fell ill. One of her anxieties was that she would be unable to have intercourse when her husband was improved.

On examination she was a tall well-built woman but not overweight. She was normotensive and her general examination was satisfactory. Palpation of the abdomen was normal. On pelvic examination in the modified left lateral position the introitus and vulva appeared normal although the perineum was deficient at the site of a previous episiotomy. At rest, the posterior wall of the vagina appeared to protrude through a slightly gaping introitus. On straining however, the anterior wall descended to be followed by the appearance of a healthy cervix which protruded through the introitus but no more. There was no leakage of urine on straining or coughing. On passing a Sims speculum along the posterior wall of the vagina, straining dislocated the whole of the anterior vaginal wall downwards. On reversing the speculum, and again asking the patient to strain, there was no descent of the posterior vaginal wall at any level. On bimanual examination, the uterus was of normal size and very mobile. It was axial in position. The cervix was elongated so that the appearance of the cervix at the introitus did not represent true uterine descent although there was clearly some. The adnexae were normal.

Questions

How would you summarize your findings?

The patient presents with symptoms of prolapse sufficient to interfere with her day to day activities. On examination she has a uterovaginal prolapse. There is first to second degree uterine prolapse and a large urethrocystocele. There is no demonstrable posterior wall prolapse but the perineum is deficient.

What treatment would you advise this woman to have?

In the first instance I would suggest that we try to control the prolapse with a ring pessary.

Why?

It is probable that the heavy work involved with looking after her husband has precipitated the prolapse in the first place. Her husband is still unwell and she continues to nurse him. If an operation were performed now, and she returned home to that situation, then the chances of a recurrent prolapse would be high. The first definitive operation is likely to be the most successful and it should therefore be undertaken only in the most favourable circumstances. The prolapse is not gross and there are no symptoms of incontinence. The chances of achieving control are good. Furthermore, she complains of backache and ascribes this to the prolapse. This may not be the cause of her backache which is more likely to be related to her increased activity. Control of the prolapse with a ring pessary should identify the scope of symptomatic relief that might be expected from surgery.

For what other reasons might you resort to a pessary rather than surgery?

If the patient is considered too frail for surgery. This should only exceptionally be the case because the usual concern for such patients is the anaesthetic risk and most vaginal procedures can be accomplished under epidural or spinal block. The patient may not entertain a hysterectomy in some cases when a vaginal hysterectomy might be the procedure of choice. In pregnancy a pessary can support the enlarging uterus until such time as it is large enough to support itself above the pelvic brim. In the same way it can be replaced after confinement until involution is complete and lactation discontinued before embarking on surgery. A pessary can be used during the interim to control the prolapse if further pregnancies are planned quickly. If the interval is long then repair of the prolapse is indicated. The patient should then understand, that in a subsequent pregnancy, she might be delivered abdominally to safeguard the repair. In the event of decubital ulceration on a prolapse of long standing, reduction of the prolapse and its support by a ring pessary will promote healing.

Are there any problems with the use of ring and other pessaries?

Yes, neglect! Sometimes the patient is so pleased with the relief that a pessary can bring that she forgets that a surgical procedure has been suggested. Because she feels well she then sees little purpose in attending the clinic for regular review. The result can be ulceration of the vaginal skin with superinfection. In addition, such ulcers can undergo malignant transformation. Neglected rings can become incarcerated within the vagina requiring a general anaesthetic for their removal. Fistula formation into the bladder or rectum can occur. The rings should be checked every 3 to 4 months. The old ring should be removed and the vagina carefully inspected for ulceration. If all is clear a new ring can be inserted. With time, some patients find that with the shrinkage of tissue the prolapse becomes self supporting and the ring is no longer required. If inflammation is detected then replacement of the pessary should be deferred until healing is complete. This can often be promoted by the application of oestrogen cream.

Let us assume that the patient elects to proceed with surgery, what operation would you advise in this case?

I would advise a vaginal hysterectomy. Although the patient's menses are satisfactory she is 45 years of age with a grown up family. The procedure allows also for the inspection of the ovaries. There is descent of the uterus although not as much as one would suspect by seeing the cervix presenting at the vulva. A final decision on the precise operation could be deferred until the patient was on the operating table. However, an assessment of the vaginal capacity with a view to coitus is best made with the patient conscious. I would combine the vaginal hysterectomy with an anterior colporrhaphy.

Would you take any particular steps during the execution of this operation?

One complication of the operation is shortening of the anterior vaginal wall. For this reason particular care must be taken to remove the minimum of vaginal skin during the anterior colporrhaphy and to use interrupted sutures for the closure of the anterior suture line. The operation also has a reputation for recurrence in the form of an enterocele. When, during the operation, the peritoneum of the pouch of Douglas is opened any enterocele sac or redundant peritoneum should be excised. Later it is essential that once the uterus has been taken and the pedicles secured the ligatures securing the combined uterosacral/cardinal ligament pedicles are tied together and then put on stretch by pulling the ligatures anteriorly. This makes the medial edges of the uterosacral ligaments more prominent posterior to the dissection enabling them to be mattressed together with additional sutures, thus closing off the base of the pouch of Douglas and closing the potential gap for the development of an enterocele.

Would you undertake a posterior repair?

Posterior colpoperineorrhaphy is not an essential part of the procedure. It can cause retention of urine after surgery, and cause coital difficulties subsequently. However, in this case the perineum is deficient and the introitus is gaping. I would assess the introitus before surgery and undertake a small posterior repair.

Do you employ any specific pre- or postoperative measures?

Vault haematoma and infection are known complications of the procedure. Large accumulations will drain down from the vault. I believe that prophylactic antibiotics reduce the morbidity associated with the operation and I prescribe metronidazole suppositories from the time of the premedication until 48 h after surgery. Suprapubic drainage of the bladder is established in theatre before the patient returns to the ward and trimethoprin prescribed until the catheter is removed. I do not prescribe s.c. heparin prophylactically unless the patient is obese or has a history of thromboembolic disease. The patient however should wear anti-embolic stockings and be mobilized as quickly as possible.

What other surgical technique could be employed for this patient?

A Manchester repair.

What do you mean by that?

The definition can vary from text to text. Basically, the operation combines anterior colporrhaphy with amputation of the cervix and posterior colporrhaphy. The key to the operation is the division of the cardinal and uterosacral ligaments at their insertion into the cervix before amputation of the cervix and then the suturing of the cut ligaments in front of the cervical stump. This manoeuvre has the effect of essentially shortening the cardinal ligaments thus elevating the vault and anteverting the uterus from its axial position in association with prolapse. The anterior wall is also lengthened.

It would be suitable in this case where elongation of the cervix is a feature and actual descent of the uterus is not gross.

Discussion

Vault inversion following vaginal or abdominal hysterectomy remains a difficult problem to solve. Consequently a number of procedures are offered none of which is entirely satisfactory in all cases. The first consideration is whether coitus is to continue. If this is not a requirement then a vigorous anterior and posterior colporrhaphy with excision of any enterocele and narrowing of the vagina may be successful. A Le Fort procedure with the obliteration of the vagina by apposing the anterior and posterior vagina walls can control the inversion but the resultant distortion of the anatomy can affect the functioning of the internal sphincter resulting in urinary sphincter incontinence.

When sexual function is to be conserved an abdominal route is usually adopted. The procedures described depend on the anchoring of the vaginal vault to the promontory of the sacrum. A variety of materials are used to bridge the gap. Mersilene mesh or strips of external oblique aponeurosis have been utilized. These techniques appear to be more successful in preventing recurrence than the older method of securing the vaginal angles to the residual round ligaments on each side. A vaginal procedure is described commencing with the identification of any enterocele and its excision. The dissection is carried laterally displacing the rectum backwards and medially affording access to the sacrospinous ligament. The vault is then secured to the ligament close to the spine before completing the operation with a colpoperineorrhaphy.

Comment

When presenting a case of prolapse it is important to pay attention to the general examination. Prolapse need not only ensue when the supporting structures become weakened but also when the intra-abdominal pressure is raised. Prolapse can be the first sign of an intra-abdominal mass. The author experienced a case where the patient presented with a total procidentia. She was obese but on examination it was clear that there were large bilateral ovarian masses. These were secondary to a small carcinoma of the breast of which the patient was completely unaware.

The demonstration of the physical signs in these cases should be polished and purposeful. Prolapse is best demonstrated with the patient in the left lateral position. The candidate must be totally competent in the use of the Simms speculum and the vaginal elevator. Good lighting is essential and the candidate can call on an attendant to assist in the positioning of the patient if necessary. A clear view is essential if there is a significant posterior vaginal wall prolapse and the coexistence of an enterocele with a rectocele is to be recognized. The elevator can be used to good effect lifting the anterior wall forward as the Simms speculum is slowly withdrawn from the posterior fornix to the introitus releasing first the enterocele and then a rectocele if present. If the prolapse is purely vaginal and considerable it may not be possible to visualize the cervix using the Simms speculum. It is quite acceptable to pass a Cusco speculum subsequently in order to complete the examination. If the patient has been lying down for any length of time the prolapse may reduce and the signs be difficult to elicit. This may also be because the patient is shy about straining with any effort for fear of passing flatus. The anus should therefore be supported by the observer when asking the patient to bear down. If this does not work then it is in order to suggest to the examiner that the patient be asked to stand by the bed and strain down to maximize the descent of any prolapse. During this manoeuvre the patient should be afforded every consideration as she may find this technique very much more embarrassing than the usual examination. There is no single correct way to conduct the examination under these circumstances. The examination is only complete when all the necessary and available information has been obtained. To do this may require a degree of extemporization by the candidate. The examiner will judge the result on the information gained and the sympathetic handling of the patient.

Cases of genital prolapse frequently feature in the clinical examination. In such cases great emphasis is placed on the execution of the clinical examination. Much of the viva component is likely to be concerned with the practical aspects of surgery and the candidate's own experience and management.

Case 11

The 21-year-old patient presented in the antenatal clinic giving a history of a last recorded period 22 weeks before. This was her fifth pregnancy. Her husband was employed as a plasterer and they lived in a three bedroomed council house. The pregnancy was unplanned. After each of her previous pregnancies the appropriate agencies, GP, midwife, health visitor and social worker had all tried to encourage the couple to utilize some form of contraception but without success. She was symptom free and resigned to another pregnancy but on this occasion was requesting a sterilization procedure after delivery. She received a lot of support from her family and the social services. The medical history and family history were unremarkable. Her cycle was regular, 5/28. She smoked ten cigarettes per day but did not admit to taking alcohol. The obstetric history was as follows.

At 16 years of age she presented in the casualty department with acute appendicitis at 30 weeks gestation. The pregnancy had been concealed. Appendicectomy was performed. Isoxsuprine hydrochloride was given intravenously after surgery. She recovered well and the pregnancy continued uneventfully. Labour supervened spontaneously at term and she was delivered normally of a female infant weighing 2920 g.

At 17 years of age she had a twin pregnancy. She became anaemic during pregnancy and was admitted for an intravenous infusion of iron dextran at 36 weeks. Within 24 h she established spontaneous labour and was delivered of dissimilar (although female) twins. Both twins presented by the breech and required assisted breech delivery under epidural anaesthesia. They weighed 2090 g and 1900 g.

At 19 years of age she had an uneventful singleton pregnancy, with a normal delivery at term of a male infant weighing 3420 g. The first stage lasted 2 h and 20 min.

At 20 years of age she had a twin pregnancy. She was well throughout pregnancy with the spontaneous onset of labour at 37 weeks. The first twin presented by the head and was delivered normally. The second twin developed a compound presentation. Attempts to correct the situation per vaginum were unsuccessful and fetal distress developed. The second twin was delivered by caesarean section. The baby was delivered through a transverse lower segment uterine incision. The puerperium appears to have been straight forward, there being no history of fever or the prescription of antibiotics. The babies were again female binovular twins. They weighed 2630 g and 2125 g at birth. Twin 2 developed a transient Erb's palsy which resolved within a few days. This baby's subsequent development has been normal.

Her expected date of delivery was established as near as possible by ultrasound measurements of the singleton fetus at booking. The estimated date of delivery is 3 weeks earlier than her recorded dates would suggest. This margin has been confirmed by two subsequent ultrasound examinations at 28 and 32 weeks. She is now at 37 weeks on assessed dates.

On examination she weighs 57.5 kg and is well with no clinical signs of anaemia. A systemic examination is normal apart from the midline caesarean section scar. She is normotensive, blood pressure 175/75 mmHg. The uterine size is consistent with a 37 weeks gestation with a symphysial-fundal height of 36 cm and an abdominal girth measured at the umbilicus of 38 inches. The single fetus occupies a longitudinal lie with the head presenting. Three-fifths of the fetal head are palpable above the pelvic brim. There is a normal amount of amniotic fluid present. The fetal back is on the left and the fetal heart is clearly auscultated at 140 beats per min. There is no tenderness or discomfort on palpating the lower segment.

Questions

From the history what do you perceive as the principal issues in this patient's management?

Grande multiparity in a young patient
The establishment of the expected date of delivery
The mode of delivery after previous caesarean section
Sterilization in a young patient

This patient was only 16 years of age when she had her first pregnancy. From your experience what particular problems are associated with this group of patients?

Approximately 20% of women in this country experience a pregnancy by the age of 20 years and therefore the problem is common. A third of such pregnancies are terminated with the risk of the morbidity associated with such procedures. The dangers of teenage pregnancy have been overemphasized in the past and providing that antenatal care is optimal the attendant risks can be minimized. Unfortunately, as illustrated in this case, the teenager tends to present late in the clinic and often attends the clinic infrequently. Hence anaemia which is common may be missed or as occurred in this patient's second pregnancy detected too late for correction before delivery. The caesarean section rate usually approximates to that for all primigravidae in the background population. The perinatal mortality in this group is increased largely as a result of pre-eclampsia (which may fulminate early) and preterm labour. Particularly if the mother is unsupported these children are more likely to be subjected to physical abuse or psychosocial deprivation. Despite the experience of an unplanned pregnancy contraceptive advice is often ineffectual.

How would you deliver this patient?

Almost certainly by vaginal delivery. The indication for the caesarean section in the previous pregnancy was fetal distress and malpresentation and therefore 'non-recurrent'. The malpresentation of the second twin was not caused by macrosomia or cephalopelvic disproportion. She has already been delivered of a singleton fetus weighing 3420 g, after a short labour. Before committing myself to any decision I would request details of the procedure from the hospital concerned. The delivery of what sounded like a shoulder presentation can be difficult even with a small baby and sometimes the incision in the lower segment may extend or even be modified to encroach on the upper segment. If there were any doubts then a repeat caesarean section would be indicated. There was no history of postpartum genital tract infection that might have threatened the normal healing of the uterine scar. The mother has not expressed any preference for the mode of delivery but an operative delivery carries with it a greater risk of maternal mortality and morbidity.

Would you wish to undertake any further investigations before coming to this conclusion?

I would perform a clinical assessment of the pelvis to evaluate its shape and to exclude unfavourable features such as prominent ischial spines, flattened sacrum or hooked sacrum, reduced sacrospinous ligaments or reduced outlet diameters. It would also assist in determining whether the head of the fetus would engage in labour. If there were any concern then perhaps an erect lateral pelvimetry would be helpful together with an ultrasound assessment of fetal weight.

What is your preferred abdominal incision for caesarean section?

A low Pfannenstiel incision. The incision heals rapidly and well and is cosmetically acceptable to the patient. Dissection of the tissue planes can lead to ooze and haematoma formation but this disadvantage usually can be prevented by draining the wound for the first 24 h.

Why then do you think this patient had a subumbilical midline incision?

The indication for surgery was fetal distress with malpresentation. Speed of entry was therefore a major consideration as was access. It was always possible that it might have proved difficult to extract the fetus through a lower segment incision or the findings may have dictated a classical caesarean section.

Would you use oxytocin to induce labour or augment labour in such cases?

The coexistence of a pregnancy complication, sufficient to warrant induction of labour, and a previous caesarean section scar indicates a repeat caesarean section. Although the risk to the fetus of a trial of scar may be minimized it is still greater than for labour with an intact uterus. This risk is in addition to the factor indicating induction of labour.

Once the decision has been made that it is reasonable for this uterus to function in spontaneous labour then there is no logical reason why uterine contractions should not be augmented when ineffectual. In this case the infusion must be commenced cautiously as she is a grande multiparae with a record of short labour. The baby's fetal heart should be monitored electronically throughout labour. The mother should be attended at all times and her vital signs (blood pressure and pulse) recorded at 15 min intervals. The attendant should be conversant with the signs of impending scar dehiscence or rupture. Ideally an intrauterine catheter should be inserted to quantitatively record the intrauterine pressure generated by contractions in order to avoid uterine hypertonus.

What are the signs of impending dehiscence or rupture?

1. A rising maternal pulse
2. Serosanguinous or bloody loss per vaginum
3. Tenderness over the lower segment scar
4. Fetal heart rate anomalies
5. Apparent cessation of labour or failure to progress despite good uterine activity
6. Haematuria

Discussion

'Once a caesarean always a caesarean' was not unreasonable when first introduced as a rule of thumb in the early decades of the century. The prime concern was for the survival of the mother and the fetus was essentially a passive participant in parturition and only evoked intervention in its own right after delivery. Caesarean section for reasons other than major disproportion were rare and the classical operation was the operation performed.

With the universal adoption of the lower segment operation the surgical risks were reduced and intervention on behalf of the fetus became commonplace. Consequently, the number of women undergoing caesarean section for the first time increased and routine repeat sections contributed further to an accelerating number of surgical deliveries. To break this spiral, trial of labour with the scarred uterus has been advocated in order to achieve vaginal delivery after previous caesarean section. This is only valid if such management, albeit with the inherent risk of uterine rupture, is shown to carry minimal risk to mother or baby and that repeat caesarean section is associated with at least an equivalent risk.

No properly controlled randomized trials have been instituted to compare the results of elective caesarean section and trial of uterine scar. Of women allowed to undergo labour after a previous caesarean section 55% will achieve a vaginal delivery. The incidence of dehiscence discovered at elective caesarean section in such cases is similar to that found following a trial of scar (0.8–1.5%). Blood transfusion, pneumonia, pyelonephritis, wound infection, anaesthetic complications, septicaemia and thrombo-embolic complications are less common in those women who achieve a vaginal delivery following low transverse caesarean section. The estimated maternal fatality rate for caesarean section is 45 per 100 000 caesarean sections, four times the risk of vaginal delivery. Elective repeat caesarean operation is associated with a reduced risk to the mother but nevertheless is double that of vaginal delivery. Since 1970 the Reports on Confidential Enquiries into Maternal Deaths in England and Wales have recorded 43 deaths from uterine rupture. Five only of these cases were the result of scar rupture. Despite the increasing tendency to try for a vaginal delivery after a previous caesarean section there have been no recorded deaths from scar dehiscence in the past two reports (1979–1981, 1982–1984).

Perinatal mortality and morbidity rates are similar in the two groups but the two groups of babies are not strictly comparable as, very premature, abnormal or dead fetuses will tend to be delivered vaginally. Babies born by caesarean section are more likely to suffer from surfactant deficiency than babies delivered by caesarean section after labour has started or babies delivered vaginally.

The selection of patients for a trial of labour has depended on a number of factors:

1. The indication for the initial caesarean section. It has been the custom to allocate the indications into 'none recurrent', e.g. fetal distress, breech, APH, pre-eclampsia and 'recurrent', e.g.

cephalopelvic disproportion or failed trial of labour. The latter are considered by some to contraindicate a trial of scar. Each case must be considered on its merits, although the outcome is most likely to be a vaginal delivery when the initial indication had been a breech presentation. In most series, half the patients have delivered vaginally when the caesarean operation had been undertaken for disproportion, dystocia or failure to progress. Subsequent uterine rupture when reported, has been associated predominately with the non-recurrent group, where the lower segment had been relatively unformed, compared with the situation following a full trial of labour where the lower segment would have been well formed.

2. Higher rates of vaginal delivery are achieved in those women who have had a vaginal delivery before.
3. Gestational age at previous section. With advances in neonatal care, there is increased pressure to deliver small babies in peril between 26 and 30 weeks by caesarean section. These operations are frequently difficult and often the lower segment is poorly developed. Vertical incisions may have to be employed, and are recommended by some, to minimize trauma to the fetus. The vertical incision does represent an increased hazard in subsequent pregnancies and until the picture becomes clearer it would be wise to regard transverse incisions in early gestation with equal circumspection.
4. Integrity of the scar: hysterosalpingography was once employed to evaluate the healing of the lower segment incision. The configuration of an X-ray image does not identify the condition of the scar or how it will perform in a subsequent labour. Because wound infection is associated with poor quality healing in abdominal wounds, genital tract infection following caesarean section is considered to be a contraindication to an attempted vaginal delivery.
5. Configuration of the uterine incision: the classical caesarean section scar is more likely to rupture and may do so suddenly during pregnancy before the onset of labour or planned repeat operation. Rupture of the classical scar is associated with severe abdominal pain and collapse whereas the rupture of the transverse scar tends to be more silent. The development of pain is variable and the rapid development of shock unusual. The transverse scar is less likely to give way before the onset of labour. Vertical incisions in the lower segment are best considered like hysterotomy scars as behaving like the classical incision.

6. More than one previous caesarean section: the number of cases described in the literature is small but the evidence would suggest that such women could be treated as women with only one caesarean section.
7. Multiple pregnancy following a previous caesarean section should not be taken as an absolute indication for repeat operation providing the first twin presents by the vertex.

In summary, a trial of labour following caesarean operation can be recommended for women fulfilling the following criteria: one low transverse caesarean section incision, a singleton vertex presentation, and no absolute indication for caesarean section in the current pregnancy. A history of classical, low vertical, hysterotomy, or unknown uterine incision remains a contra-indication to a trial of labour.

Comment

Even an apparently straightforward case can yield rich ground for the examiner. If the examination and history of the current pregnancy is normal there is always the past obstetric, medical or family history to refer to, hence the referral to teenage pregnancy. Later the candidate's view on the management of the case is solicited. Whatever the examiner's personal view might be about the wisdom of obtaining an X-ray pelvimetry under the circumstances, the candidate's response is reasonable and defendable. The examiner's questioning revealed that although the candidate preferred a low transverse approach for caesarean section he was nevertheless aware that an alternative incision was desirable under certain circumstances. Flexibility and adaptability must not be confused with uncertainty and examiners will favour the former but not the latter. The questioning to this point was fairly predictable. A more contentious area was entered when the discussion explored the place of induction of labour in the presence of a previous caesarean section scar. Individuals (including examiners) may hold strong (and opposing) views on the subject. Providing that the candidate is aware of the debate and the arguments then he is in a position to substantiate his own stand and discuss the opposing view.

Outcome

The patient presented in spontaneous labour at 39 weeks gestation. As agreed with the patient antenatally, an epidural anaesthetic was administered. After a labour of 5 h and 45 min she was delivered normally of a male infant weighing 3700 g. Depot Provera was administered for contraception at the time of her discharge home and a laparoscopic sterilization performed 3 months later.

Further reading

DEWHURST, C. J. (1957) The ruptured caesarean section scar. *Journal of Obstetrics and Gynaecology of the British Empire*, **64**, 113–118

GILBERT, L., SAUNDERS, N. and SHARP, F. (1988) The management of multiple pregnancy in women with a lower-segment caesarean scar. Is a repeat caesarean section really the 'safe' option? *British Journal of Obstetrics and Gynaecology*, **95**, 1312–1316

OSBOURNE, G. K. (1981) Obstetric outcome of teenage pregnancy. *British Journal of Obstetrics and Gynaecology*, **88**, 215–221

PETITTI, D. B., CEFALO, R. C., SHAPIRO S. and WHALLEY, P. (1982) In hospital maternal mortality in the United States: Time trends and relation to method of delivery. *Obstetrics and Gynecology*, **59**, 6–11

Case 12

A Caucasian 30-year-old single secretary was referred to the out-patient department because of increasing hair growth over her face and arms for 12 months. Over the same period she had gained 4 kg in weight. Her menarche had been at the age of 13 years and her cycle had been regular, 5/26, until 6 months before when her cycle had become very irregular and she had missed periods. The exact dates were not available for inspection. She had a regular boyfriend and was sexually active. They used barrier contraception. She had noticed some deepening of her voice. There were no other specific gynaecological symptoms. Her past medical and family history were unremarkable and she was on no medication.

On examination she presented as a thin woman weighing 50 kg and standing 1.6 m tall. There was obvious hirsutism with abnormal hair growth involving the upper lip, chin, breasts, arms, legs and trunk. There was no recession of the temporal hair line. The Ferriman and Gallwey score was 19. The breasts were small but Tanner V. Her abdominal examination was normal apart from the male escutcheon; there were no striae. There was some clitoromegaly. The vulva, vagina and cervix were normal. The uterus was normal sized, anteverted and mobile. The left adnexum was normal. On the right the ovary was palpable approximately three times normal size, and mobile. Rectal examination confirmed the findings.

Questions

What are the most likely conditions to cause these features?

The patient complains about excess facial and body terminal hair, i.e. hirsutism, but there are two features in the history and examination which suggest actual virilism. The deepening voice, and the suggestion of clitoromegaly imply the presence of excess circulating androgens which have precipitated the development of masculine traits. Other signs of virilism include frontal baldness, breast atrophy, and the development of a male body habitus.

The presence of virilism would suggest congenital adrenal hyperplasia, a tumour of the adrenal, or a masculinizing tumour of the ovary. Other conditions to consider are idiopathic hirsutism (racial and familial), polycystic ovary syndrome, Cushing's syndrome, hyperprolactinaemia, hypothyroidism, and the use of drugs such as phenytoin, minoxidil, Mixogen®, danazol and diazoxide.

What would be your initial investigations?

1. A pelvic ultrasound to confirm or exclude the ovarian enlargement detected on clinical examination and to possibly identify PCOS.
2. Plasma LH and FSH. A markedly raised LH (except at ovulation) or an LH to FSH ratio greater than 3.0 would suggest PCOS.
3. A 24 h urinary free cortisol is a useful screen for Cushing's syndrome. A 24 h urinary 17-oxosteroid level would indicate high circulating androgens. However, if the principal androgen is testosterone, because of its potency there may be profound clinical effects with only a marginal increase in the urinary oxosteroid excretion.
4. Plasma cortisol, testosterone, androstenedione and 17-alpha-hydroxyprogesterone. If all these are raised then the picture is very suggestive of an adrenal disfunction. If so, the elevated levels will be suppressed by the administration of dexamethasone and if, on stimulation with ACTH (Synacthen®), there is a

disproportionate rise in the 17-alpha-hydroxyprogesterone, then the diagnosis is almost certainly congenital adrenal hyperplasia with 17-hydroxylase deficiency. There will also be a corresponding increase in the urinary oxosteroid excretion.

5. Dehydroepiandrosterone (DHEA) and dehydroepiandrosterone sulphate (DHEAS) levels are raised in tumours of adrenal origin.
6. Plasma SHBG. If the level of the plasma testosterone is markedly raised ($> \times 3$) with a normal SHGB then there is a high probability of an ovarian androblastoma. Depressed levels of SHBG are a feature of PCOS.
7. Oestradiol levels are normal in PCOS but the oestrone level is raised.

Our investigations confirmed a raised serum testosterone (5.6 nmol/l), and a normal androstenedione level. The LH to FSH ratio was unremarkable. There was ACTH suppression after giving dexamethasone but the serum testosterone and androsterone remained unchanged. The thyroid function tests were normal as was the serum oestradiol. The ultrasound examination confirmed enlargement of the right ovary by a solid tumour.

Those findings would suggest that the cause of this patient's hirsutism and virilization was caused by a tumour of the right ovary.

What confirmatory investigation would you undertake?

Laparotomy. The clinical findings of a significantly enlarged ovary have been confirmed by ultrasound and the biochemical investigations support the diagnosis of some form of ovarian androblastoma. The ovary needs to be removed for histological examination. Androblastomas such as Sertoli–Leydig cell tumours (arrhenoblastomas) and hilus cell tumours mostly occur in young women and are unilateral in 90% of cases. Recurrence in the contralateral ovary is rare and therefore removal of the affected ovary only is appropriate, so that she can maintain her fertility.

Why not laparoscopy?

Laparoscopy would not carry the management much further forward. The nature of an ovarian tumour cannot be determined by its gross appearances in most instances. Endocrinologically active tumours are often small lying within the matrix of the ovary so that laparoscopic biopsy could be misleading.

What is the main drug treatment for hirsutism when there is no underlying problem to be rectified?

The giving of cyproterone acetate. This anti-androgen is effective although it can alter liver function. It is normally administered as the 'reverse sequential regimen' with ethinyloestradiol. Cyproterone acetate 50 mg daily is given between days 5 and 15 of the menstrual cycle and ethinyloestradiol 30 μg is given between days 5 and 25 of the cycle. The treatment is well tolerated although there can be some weight gain. Cyproterone acetate competes with androgens at the end organ and the oestrogen boosts the levels of SHBG reducing the amount of free testosterone in the plasma. The drugs need to be given for 6–12 months before an effect will be seen on hair cover. Anti-androgens lessen hair cover but not hair colour which is often a significant problem best treated by cosmetic measures. Cyproterone acetate will cause feminization of a male fetus if administered in pregnancy. Pregnancy should be excluded before treatment and conception delayed for at least 3 months after cessation of therapy.

Discussion

Tanner's scale is used to define stages in breast development:

Stage 1 Prepubertal stage before development has occurred.
Stage 2 Breast bud beneath the nipple can be seen and palpated.
Stage 3 Breast grows and becomes more rounded resembling the adult breast but significantly smaller.
Stage 4 Nipple and areolar now project forward in front of the breast as a secondary mound.
Stage 5 Full adult form and size of the breast.

The description of hair cover is often very subjective and over a period of time and treatment the patient's perceptions of change and those of her attendants may differ. The Ferriman and Gallwey Score is an attempt to quantify the amount of terminal hair encountered during the physical examination. Eleven body areas are assessed: the upper lip, chin, chest, upper back, lower back, upper abdomen, lower abdomen, arm, forearm, thigh and leg. Each area is assigned a score of one to four depending on the density and distribution of terminal hair at those locations. A score of eight or more is consistent with a diagnosis of hirsutism, a score of 12 or more strongly suggests an androblastoma as a cause.

Oral contraceptives may be beneficial as a first line of treatment for simple hirsutism when ovarian dysfunction is suspected. The oestrogen reduces gonadotrophin levels lowering LH and ovarian androgen production is decreased. The oestrogen also increases the production of SHBG by the liver reducing the fraction of free and therefore biologically active testosterone. The progesterone reduces circulating ACTH and consequently DHEA and DHEAS levels are reduced. Progesterone probably also competes at the level of the hair follicle with testosterone.

Where the cause of the hirsutism lies in the adrenal gland, steroids (dexamethasone 0.75 mg/day) can be effective. The patient, however, is subjected to all the risks of adrenal suppression. Glucocorticoids and oral contraceptives can be used in combination to produce a synergistic effect.

Spironolactone, the aldosterone antagonist, decreases the testosterone production rate and competitively competes with testosterone at the hair follicle.

Cyproterone acetate has been described in the presentation above.

Cosmetic techniques are indicated in mild cases and when treatment has achieved some effect. If the hair growth is slight nothing more than bleaching may be required. Superfluous hair may be removed by the use of depilatory wax, shaving or pumice stone but these treatments require repetition. Shaving does not encourage stronger growth of hair. Electrolysis is painful and very expensive and again is not a permanent cure. Furthermore it may leave scars. New chemical depilatories are useful in some cases and harmless.

Androblastomas are tumours composed of Sertoli cells, Leydig cells or the precursors of either, alone or in combination. These tumours were originally referred to as arrhenoblastomas which implied that they were inevitably virilizing. This is not the case and rarely they can cause oestrogenism. Androblastoma is preferred because the term indicates that the tumours reflect phases in the development of the male gonad.

Outcome

Laparotomy was performed and the enlarged right ovary removed. The ovary contained a well-differentiated Sertoli–Leydig cell tumour (arrhenoblastoma). Within 4 days the patient's testosterone levels had fallen to normal limits. Subsequently normal menstruation supervened. Her hirsutism almost completely resolved but the voice change and slight clitoromegaly remained unchanged.

Further reading

DECHERNEY, A. H. (1981) The investigation and treatment of hirsutism. In *Progress in Obstetrics and Gynaecology* (ed J. Studd), Vol 1, Churchill Livingstone, London, Ch. 21.

HAMMERSTEIN, J., MECKIES, J., LEO-ROSSBERG, I., MOLTZ, L. and ZIELSKE F. (1975) Use of cyproterone acetate in the treatment of acne, hirsutism and virilism. *Journal of Steroid Biochemistry*, **6**, 827–836

UNDERHILL, R. and DEWHURST, J. (1979) Further clinical experience in the treatment of hirsutism with cyproterone acetate. *British Journal of Obstetrics and Gynaecology*, **86**, 139–141

Case 13

The 19-year-old patient lived with her boyfriend in bed and breakfast accommodation provided by the local council. Both were unemployed. The patient had been adopted and had no knowledge of her family's medical history. This pregnancy was her first. She had only a vague notion as to the date of her last menstrual period. Several appointments had been made to see her in the clinic after receiving a booking letter from her GP. The appointment that resulted in her first visit had been asked for by a victim support group. When seen, clinical examination suggested a 20-week pregnancy and this was confirmed by an ultrasound examination. On examination nothing abnormal was recorded except that she was a 'poor specimen' weighing 49.2 kg. Routine investigations were normal. Her only complaint was that she felt tired. It transpired that she had not attended the clinic because she could not afford the fares. She was also changing her domicile frequently. Her antenatal care was arranged at the hospital to facilitate the involvement of the medical social worker in this obvious case of need. Her antenatal care progressed normally to 35 weeks when she complained that she felt exhausted, and had experienced two episodes of loss of vision and hearing in the last 2 weeks. The episodes had lasted for 15 min. There was no loss of consciousness. Of greatest concern to her was an increasing tendency for her legs to give way for no apparent reason, causing her to fall to the floor. She could get up immediately but her legs felt 'wobbly'. This had last happened at a supermarket checkout and had caused her extreme embarrassment.

She is now at 36 weeks gestation as determined by ultrasound and weighs 53 kg. Her BP is 115/70 mmHg. She looks pale but is not clinically anaemic. Her face is to a degree expressionless but symmetrical. There is bilateral ptosis more pronounced on the right than on the left. The pupils are equal and symmetrical. Pupillary and accommodatory reflexes are intact. There is no compensatory over activity of the frontalis muscle. The examination of the cranial nerves is normal. There appears to be symmetrical wasting of both forearms and quadriceps. Peripheral reflexes are intact. Power of grip is not reduced in either hand but there appears to be some difficulty in relaxing the grip. There is no sensory loss demonstrable. Her gait is normal. The optic fundi are normal.

The uterine size is compatible with a 36-week gestation. A single fetus presents by the vertex; the head is not engaged, three-fifths remaining palpable above the pelvic brim. There is the impression of excess liquor. The fetal heart rate is 148 beats/min and regular.

Questions

How would you propose to manage this situation?

Apart from a rather poor weight gain (4 kg in 16 weeks) the pregnancy clinically is progressing normally. The main concern is the nature of the neurological problem that has developed during the pregnancy. For this I would seek a neurological opinion to possibly diagnose the condition and to advise on suitable investigations.

What do the physical signs suggest?

The ptosis is pronounced but asymmetrical. Ptosis can occur with third nerve palsies but in this case both sides would need to be involved and as eye movements and accommodatory reflexes are intact it is unlikely that this is the cause of the ptosis. Ptosis can also result from sympathetic nerve involvement such as is seen in Horner's syndrome, but the absence of meiosis would preclude this diagnosis. Myasthenia gravis can produce a similar picture but muscular atrophy is not a feature of this condition. Tabes dorsalis is associated with bilateral partial ptosis but this is unlikely in view of the negative screening tests. Congenital ptosis is present from birth and accompanied by frontalis over action. Peripheral neuropathy would normally be associated with pain or discomfort and absent or reduced reflexes.

The picture is therefore of some form of muscular dysfunction.

Neurophysiological studies demonstrated normal nerve conduction both motor and sensory in the upper limb. An electromyogram confirmed profuse myotonic discharges and myopathic changes distally in the upper limbs. The picture is typical of myotonica dystrophica. Would you let pregnancy progress beyond term?

The only reason to deliver the baby at term would be if the baby were then judged to be at risk or if the mother's condition were likely to demand it. The pregnancy appears to be progressing normally and the baby is not compromised. The dates are also to some extent uncertain being established by rather late ultrasound at 20 weeks. I would await the spontaneous onset of labour.

How long would you be prepared to wait? Indefinitely?

There is much discussion as to whether or not pregnancy should be allowed to continue beyond 42 weeks. I recognize an increased perinatal mortality for babies delivered later than this, although the causes may be many and some not specifically related to the period of gestation. I would therefore advise induction of labour at 42 weeks. In this case there is some doubt as to precise dates, but the estimate is based on ultrasound measurement and induction is unlikely to produce a significantly preterm baby if undertaken at that time.

How would you manage the support of this patient in the future?

Myotonia dystrophica is an inherited condition. The diagnosis was only established in pregnancy. Apart from the involvement of specialists responsible for her future care, assistance with counselling should be solicited from the designated regional genetic centre . The appropriate consultant clinical geneticist can then advise on the risk to further pregnancies and the facilities available (if any) to identify an affected fetus. In the meantime the patient will need a great deal of support to come to terms with the implications of her own diagnosis and her care should continue under the immediate supervision of her consultant. The paediatrician should be alerted to the possibility of an affected child and likewise the GP informed as the picture develops. This patient has enormous social problems and the social agencies should be warned about the impending problems so that provision can be made for care and supervision after discharge from hospital.

Discussion

The terms postdate, postmature, prolonged and afterterm pregnancy are synonymous. The standard definition recommended by the WHO and FIGO for a post-term pregnancy is '42 completed weeks or more (294 days or more)'. This definition is concerned with the duration of pregnancy for the purpose of epidemiological studies. It does not of itself identify 'postmaturity' which is a clinical condition in the newborn associated with post-term pregnancy which is responsible for an increase in perinatal mortality. The key to the diagnosis is an accurate assessment of gestational age. Approximately 70% of women will provide a certain record of their last period, 20% an approximate figure and the remainder are uncertain. Uncertain dates are commoner in the more vulnerable patients, social classes 4 and 5, teenage mothers, poorly educated primipara and heavy smokers. The frequency of the natural cycle is often poorly recorded but any variation in the length of the menstrual cycle usually delays ovulation rather than advancing it. The number of patients going postdates will increase as the proportion of patients with uncertain dates or irregular cycles increases. These patients have babies that are not biologically post-term. In the same way postconceptional bleeding may be misinterpreted so that babies considered at term may be post-term. Intervention on 'dates' therefore may result in interference in a normal pregnancy. When dealing with limits of only 2 weeks' ultrasound examination in early pregnancy will not completely resolve this dilemma. Overall, 14–16% of pregnancies go post-term. The phenomenon is commoner in primigravidae. The risk of post-term delivery is doubled if the first birth was post-term.

However, in most series described the perinatal mortality rate for babies born post-term is double that at term. The perinatal mortality rate at term is the lowest for any stage in pregnancy and therefore this doubling of the rate does not imply large numbers of babies. The postmaturity 'syndrome' refers to those babies delivered with the stigmata of reduced subcutaneous fat, dry cracked skin and meconium staining . In the more severe forms birth asphyxia, respiratory distress, convulsions and fetal death may occur. Although such babies may weigh more than 2500 g they probably are growth retarded. The assumption has been made that these changes are the consequence only of the duration of the pregnancy and that they can be prevented by earlier delivery. In fact in normal pregnancies growth is sustained until delivery. Another assumption has been that all post-term pregnancies are pathological and demand intervention in order to prevent the development of the postmaturity syndrome. From earlier considerations a significant number of pregnancies diagnosed as postmature involve babies whose biological life is less than 42 weeks. Not all the deaths in post-term babies are retrievable . A quarter of the excess mortality post-term compared with term is from severe congenital malformation. As explained, women with uncertain dates inflate the numbers of the post-term pregnancies. There is evidence that the perinatal mortality associated with uncertain dates is increased at all gestations. Consequently 'postmaturity' may not be the only factor operating in this group in which case intervention on the grounds of gestational age alone would be inappropriate.

Once lethal malformation is excluded, the bulk of the fetal loss after 42 weeks occurs in labour or in the neonatal period. The principal causes of fetal death are intrapartum asphyxia with meconium or the complications of meconium aspiration in the neonatal period. Traumatic intracranial haemorrhage also accounts for neonatal loss which is only partially explained by an increase in forceps delivery for fetal distress and delay in the second stage. Early neonatal seizures are seen more commonly in babies delivered after 42 weeks than those born between 37 weeks and term. Again, the association with meconium in these babies is marked.

If the avoidance of meconium-stained liquor is the route to reducing perinatal death in post-term pregnancy then the logical step is to induce labour at term. Induction of labour from term onwards has been shown in controlled trials to reduce the incidence of meconium-stained amniotic fluid. The effect is more marked when induction takes place at term but there is some saving at 42 weeks also. Induction of labour at term would mean interference in half the population when the perinatal loss was minimal in order to reduce the risk of meconium-stained liquor in the few women whose pregnancies continue to 294 days and beyond. The answer as to the benefits of elective *versus* selective delivery at 290–294 days remains unresolved. Such an induction policy does not increase the recourse to caesarean section or instrumental vaginal delivery. If postnatal pregnancy were to carry a risk of 5 per 1000 for perinatal death then a trial of 70 000 subjects would be required to give an 80% chance of showing a 25% reduction in the perinatal mortality. The total of subjects in 12 controlled trials reviewed in 1989 (*vide infra*) was 3522 making any conclusions about the effect of induction policies on the risk of perinatal death impossible.

Faced with the problem of an otherwise normal pregnancy at 42 weeks gestation the first imperative is to check again the reliability of the expected date of delivery. A careful ultrasound of the fetus should be performed to exclude fetal abnormality. The case for or against induction at this stage has not been made. The issues should be explained to the patient allowing her to make a choice. Some reports suggest that the majority of women prefer that the pregnancy should continue normally until the onset of labour but it is the experience of particularly those who work with deprived populations that their patients are often pressing for delivery once the 'dates' are passed. An alternative might be to identify those women with meconium-stained amniotic fluid by serial amnioscopy the examination being carried out every 2 to 3 days after 42 weeks, together with fetal cardiotocography. The assessment of fetal well-being could be supplemented by recording fetal movements or ultrasound morphometry and assessment of amniotic fluid. The identification of meconium or fetal heart rate anomalies by such means would indicate delivery. Because of the concern for intrapartum anoxia and meconium inhalation as well as the increased incidence of intracranial haemorrhage there would be grounds to deliver such patients by caesarean section. At the very least induction of labour coupled with comprehensive fetal monitoring would be required.

Dystrophia myotonica (Myotonica atrophica) is an inherited disease transmitted as an autosomal dominant. Myotonia consists of prolonged contraction and slow relaxation of muscles resulting from repetitive contractions in muscle fibres after a single neural stimulus. Unlike most muscular diseases, distal muscles are more severely affected than proximal. The muscles earliest and most severely affected are those of the face (myasthenic facies, nasal speech and poor enucleation), the sternomastoids, forearms, quadriceps and the dorsiflexors of the feet so that there is a tendency to fall, unless the knee is kept well extended, and to trip. The onset is usually in the third decade, the course is progressive. Difficulty in relaxing the hand may be noticed before wasting is apparent. The patient frequently complains of tiredness and the need for sleep. Ptosis from weakness in the levator palpebrae and weakness of the other facial muscles gives the face the expressionless appearance . These patients develop cataracts. Gonadal atrophy can result in amenorrhoea.

In pregnancy the situation usually deteriorates with increasing weakness by 28 weeks. There is a high fetal loss from spontaneous abortion, preterm labour and in the neonatal period by congenital myotonic dystrophy. Hydramnios may develop. Labour may be prolonged or precipitate but the response to Syntocinon® is normal. Delay in the second stage is common because of maternal weakness and postpartum haemorrhage is frequent. Half the offspring will carry the gene. Prenatal diagnosis is possible by restriction fragment length polymorphism.

Comment

Candidates for the MRCOG have received a general medical education and have completed a preregistration appointment in medicine. Dystrophia myotonica is a rare condition and the examiners would not expect the candidate to be fully conversant with the details of this condition. However, they would expect a competent demonstration of the physical signs and a sensible interpretation of their significance.

In order to promote the obstetric dimension in an otherwise normal case the examiner may well pose a hypothetical problem (in this case prolonged pregnancy) to test the candidates knowledge and standards of management. The topic of 'post-maturity' has been the subject of recent meetings and review articles so that a candidate would be expected to hold an opinion and to justify it. Very often discussions such as this emanate from key papers which have triggered the debate. The candidate should be able to comment on the validity of the study especially if the numbers of subjects are sufficient statistically to reveal the end points sought.

Outcome

Five days post-term the patient presented on the labour ward in early labour. Her BP was 140/90 mmHg and the urine was loaded with protein (4+). Microscopy of the urine was clear. Rupture of the membranes released copious liquor thickly stained with meconium. Fetal monitoring was instituted via a scalp electrode and an epidural anaesthetic administered. Despite attempted augmentation of labour with Syntocinon, after 8 h there had been no further progress. A fetal scalp sampling was unsuccessfully attempted and the decision made to proceed to caesarean section. The procedure was straightforward and a female infant weighing 3060 g was delivered in good condition. After delivery the mother was nursed in a semi-erect position to reduce the effort of breathing. Her blood gases were consistently normal. Chest physiotherapy was administered from the outset to facilitate expectoration.

Electromyographic studies on the baby confirmed the congenital form of dystrophia myotonica. Nine months later the baby could roll over but not sit up. The facies were suggestive of myotonic dystrophy. The lower limbs were markedly hypotonic. Despite comprehensive counselling since the diagnosis of the mother, the couple were still not convinced that the child has a congenital form of the mother's illness.

Further reading

ARULKUMARAN, S., RAUFF, M., INGMARSSON, I., GIBB, D. M. F. and RATNAM, S. S. (1986) Uterine activity in myotonica dystrophica. Case report. *British Journal of Obstetrics and Gynaecology*, **93**, 634–636

CARDOZO, L., FYSH, J. and PEARCE, J. M. (1986) Prolonged pregnancy: the management debate. *British Medical Journal*, **293**, 1059–1063

CROWLEY, P. (1989) Post term pregnancy:induction or surveillance? In *Effective Care in Pregnancy and Childbirth* (eds I. Chalmers, M. Enkin and M. J. N. C. Keirse) Oxford University Press, Oxford, Ch. 47

HALL, M. H. and CARR-HILL, R. A. (1985) The significance of uncertain gestation for obstetric outcome. *British Journal of Obstetrics and Gynaecology*, **92**, 452–460

Case 14

The patient was 67 years of age and her referral to the gynaecological clinic was the culmination of a life-long history of urinary symptoms. As a child she was enuretic to the age of 16 years and thereafter was prone to nocturia three or four times each night. During the day there was no frequency, the patient passed urine only five or six times each day. On almost any exertion she was incontinent of urine. She also leaked when she had a desire to void. She was incontinent many times each day and used six sanitary towels daily for protection. When first married she was incontinent during intercourse and soon became apareunic and therefore involuntarily infertile. On occasion she felt a sensation of incomplete bladder emptying after voiding but had no other symptoms of voiding difficulty.

Her menopause had been at the age of 40 years. Ten years ago she had undergone a vaginal repair that had left her urinary symptoms completely unchanged. She was a known chronic depressive with a history of two admissions with overdoses;she had received intermittent psychotherapy for 20 years but was on no drug treatment at the time of referral. She was reticent about what specific investigations had been performed since she first came to the clinic. She was admitted 3 months ago for some 'injections into the bladder' but these did not make things better, in fact she felt that her symptoms had become worse.

On examination it was apparent that she was of markedly labile affect and cried during the interview. She was 1.62 m in height but weighed 86 kg. There were no other positive features on general examination. A neurological examination was satisfactory. The pelvic floor and anal sphincter tone were normal. Anal and bulbocavernosus reflexes were easily elicited, and sensation in the sacral dermatomes was normal.

The vulva was normal with no significant atrophy. There was no significant uterovaginal prolapse. With the patient lying supine on the couch, gross stress incontinence was demonstrable. The cervix was normal, and there was no abnormality on bimanual examination. The bladder was not clinically distended.

Questions

What is the most likely cause of this woman's urinary symptoms?

The history suggests a complicated picture. The lifelong history of urinary complaints;the history of enuresis into the teens; the failure to respond to previous bladder neck surgery;the symptoms of nocturia and urge, the large volumes of urine passed when incontinent, and to some extent her psychiatric problems and emotional lability would suggest detrusor instability. On the other hand there is a clear relationship between physical stress and incontinence and stress incontinence was readily demonstrated on clinical examination.

Whilst detrusor instability is the most likely single urodynamic abnormality here the suggestion of mixed pathology is such that it would be inappropriate to proceed without urodynamic investigation.

What investigations should be undertaken?

Midstream urine culture and microscopy. It is unlikely that urinary infection would be the cause of urinary incontinence of this severity or duration, although it might contribute to other irritative symptoms. In the presence of infection catheterization for urodynamic investigation may be uncomfortable and could in theory lead to an exacerbation of symptoms and in the elderly even septicaemia. If infection is identified it must be treated before carrying out urodynamic studies.

Cystometry. This is the investigation by which the pressure/volume relationships of the bladder are investigated. When combined with uroflowmetry it allows a full functional assessment of the lower urinary tract during both filling and voiding phases of the micturition cycle.

An intravenous urogram. This patient has a long-standing history of urinary problems and the possibility of residual renal damage by pyelonephritis is a possibility. For the same reason the plasma urea and electrolytes should be estimated. A creatinine clearance measurement would identify significantly reduced renal function. The IVU in this case might reveal previously unidentified renal tract anomalies.

Cystoscopy would exclude organic bladder mucosal pathology as a cause of urgency or trigone irritation.

Culture and microscopy of the urine was normal. The cystometry report was as follows:

The preliminary free urine flow rate was 25 ml/s with a voided volume of 100 ml and a normal flow pattern. On catheterization there was no residual urine. During bladder filling at 100 ml/min, the first sensation of bladder filling was appreciated at 130 ml, and the cystometric capacity was 420 ml. Several uninhibited contractions were evident during filling and recurred from 80 ml to capacity. The maximum amplitude of detrusor contractions was 26 cmH_2O. There were no further detrusor contractions evident on provocation. Marked stress incontinence was evident on coughing and straining, but without any associated increase in detrusor pressure. Voiding occurred by a combination of detrusor contraction and abdominal straining; peak urine flow on this occasion was 15 ml/s and she voided to completion.

What are your conclusions?

The urodynamic findings are of severe genuine stress incontinence. Low pressure detrusor instability is also present although it is possible that the detrusor contractions would have been higher if the urethra were more efficient. (The pressure developing in the bladder is a product of detrusor contraction and urethral resistance. If the urethra has a low resistance then the pressure within the bladder will be low either during voluntary voiding or during uninhibited contractions. Higher urethral resistance will produce higher detrusor pressure.)

Given the urodynamic findings how should our patient be managed?

It is generally accepted that where detrusor instability and genuine stress incontinence coexist it is best to control the uninhibited detrusor activity before undertaking surgical treatment of the bladder neck.

How would you achieve this?

The three main lines of management for detrusor instability are by pharmacological means, behaviour modification and by surgery.

Many antispasmodic drugs can be used although Pro-Banthine is the most widely used and the cheapest. Other drugs include oxybutidine, terodiline and imipramine. Cure rates of 20% and symptomatic relief rates of 50% can be anticipated. Anticholinergic side-effects are common but none of these drugs is specific to the bladder and a therapeutic response is uncommon unless some side-effects are apparent.

Several behavioural modification techniques have been described including bladder drill or retraining, biofeedback and hypnosis. These techniques are very time consuming of the therapist's time and demand patient motivation. Cure and improvement rates in the order of 80% have been reported.

The surgical management of detrusor instability consists of a number of techniques designed to partially denervate the bladder such as sacral neurectomy, cystodistention, bladder transection, vaginal denervation and injection of the trigone with phenol.

Alternatively, augmentation of the bladder capacity by caecocystoplasty or ileocystoplasty has been tried.

This patient was treated with subtrigonal phenol injections. She claimed that these had no effect but her cystometry was repeated. What do you conclude from the results?

The preliminary free urine flow rate was 40 ml/s and the voided volume was 725 ml. There was no residual on catheterization. The first sensation on bladder filling was at 360 ml and the cystometric filling capacity was 530 ml. Only minimal uninhibited detrusor capacity was evident at capacity with a single detrusor contraction measuring only 6 cmH_2O. Severe stress incontinence was demonstrable once more. Voiding occurred by low amplitude detrusor contraction, and again the flow rate was in excess of 40 ml/s with a maximum voiding pressure of only 4 cmH_2O.

Her detrusor instability appears to have been controlled with a significant increase in her functional and cystometric bladder capacity and a reduction in the number and magnitude of uninhibited contractions. Genuine stress incontinence remains severe.

In the light of these results should bladder neck surgery be considered?

It is sometimes stated that in the presence of detrusor instability or a combined picture of instability and stress incontinence that surgery is best avoided. The fear is aggravation of the instability component after surgery or the fact that the patient will still be left with the symptoms of detrusor instability. However, in patients where stress incontinence is the major element of their symptomatology bladder neck surgery is appropriate providing that they accept that surgery is aimed at relieving the symptom of stress incontinence and that residual frequency and urgency may persist. The concern here is the considerable functional overlay that the patient exhibits and the fact that despite objective evidence of an improvement in her bladder function her perception has been that matters have become worse.

What surgical approaches could you adopt and which would you choose?

The evidence is now good that suprapubic procedures carry better prospects for cure than a purely vaginal approach. In a patient with no uterovaginal prolapse and who has had a previous unsuccessful vaginal procedure, there can be little argument that a suprapubic procedure is to be preferred. Colposuspension probably carries the best overall prognosis for cure, although for the procedure to be technically satisfactory an adequate vaginal capacity and mobility are required. These requirements may be lacking in those patients with marked atrophic vaginal changes, a past history of vaginal surgery, those who have had radiotherapy and those who are simply nulliparous. For these patients a suburethral sling procedure or one of the more recent 'needle suspension procedures' are probably the techniques of first choice. However, sling procedures have been consistently reported to be associated with an increased voiding difficulty after surgery. Urodynamic studies confirm raised voiding pressures and decreased flow rates in the longer term after surgery. Needle suspensions such as the Stamey endoscopic bladder neck suspension do not appear to be so obstructive in general. Furthermore, needle suspension procedures involve a shorter operating time and a lower postoperative morbidity and are better suited to the older patient or the more physically frail. I would undertake a Stamey bladder neck suspension.

Discussion

While the symptom of stress incontinence may be present in women with any abnormality of lower urinary tract function, the physical sign of stress incontinence is generally held to be reasonably specific for the condition of genuine stress incontinence (urethral sphincter weakness). Several authors have suggested that leakage occurring exactly coincident with a rise in intra-abdominal pressure correlates with the diagnosis of genuine stress incontinence, whereas that occurring after a slight delay, or persisting after the intra-abdominal pressure has returned to normal, may reflect cough or stress induced detrusor contractions. However, it has been shown that during a series of coughs the urethra undergoes a process of progressive relaxation or fatigue. Patients with mild genuine stress incontinence may not leak when asked to cough only once but may do so after four or five closely repeated increases in intra-abdominal pressure, without any coexistent increase in detrusor pressure. It is also well to remember that up to three-quarters of women with voiding dysfunction and residual urine may also demonstrate the physical sign of stress incontinence.

Techniques of bladder investigation vary in terms of the route of access used to fill the bladder, the filling medium used, the temperature of the medium, the method and rate of bladder filling, the type of filling and pressure monitoring catheters, the pressure transducers used, and the amplification and recording systems employed. All the systems should allow an assessment of the detrusor response to filling and provocation, the efficiency of the detrusor during voiding, and the reserve power of the detrusor to overcome obstruction, the competence of the urethral sphincter to withstand increases in the intra-abdominal pressure, and the resistance of the urethra to urine flow. In some units cystometry is combined with simultaneous radiological screening in the form of a videocystourethrogram (VCU). This gives additional information including the presence of vesicoureteric reflux, urogenital fistulae, the siting of diverticula, the position and mobility of the bladder base in the face of voiding or increases in intra-abdominal pressure and the localization of any obstruction. Many units have considered the VCU to represent the 'gold standard' of urodynamic investigation but it is very expensive and the evidence would seem to be that in the absence of overt neurological disease it has little to offer over routine dual channel subtracted cystometry.

Intravenous urography has a specific role where congenital anomalies or ureteric fistulae are suspected and where voiding dysfunction has been proven on previous urodynamic investigation. The latter is associated with ureteric reflux and the risk of renal damage.

Conclusions regarding the function of the lower urinary tract based on endoscopic findings alone are frequently fallacious. Unless there are other features in the history to indicate its use endoscopy should probably be restricted to those cases with bladder pain, hypersensitive bladders or those with proven voiding dysfunction.

The role of urethral pressure measurement in the investigation of urinary incontinence has been the subject of perhaps more debate than any other investigation. Although the differentiation of patients with genuine stress incontinence from those with efficient sphincter function is certainly possible by the combined use of resting and stress urethral pressure profilometry (UPP), the role of this technique in clinical practice remains unproven.

Outcome

At first the patient was treated with Pro-Banthine. The dose was increased from 15 mg three times daily to 45 mg three times daily over a period of 6 weeks with no improvement. Oxybutinin also failed to provide symptomatic benefit.

She was then admitted to hospital for bladder drill and supportive psychotherapy. She was found to be voiding hourly with regular incontinence between voiding. It was suggested that she initially void more frequently to offset this problem but she was incontinent whenever she rose from her chair.

She was them admitted for cystourethroscopy under a general anaesthetic. There was no intravesical abnormality, and 6 ml of 6% phenol was injected midway between the bladder neck and the ureteric orifices on each side of the bladder base. A day later when the catheter was removed she complained that her incontinence was worse although urodynamic studies indicated that her bladder irritability was much improved although her stress incontinence remained severe.

Finally she underwent a Stamey endoscopic bladder neck suspension. At follow-up she was looking and feeling a 'new woman'. She voided only two or three times each day and there was only occasional nocturia. There was no urgency, urgency incontinence or stress incontinence. The urinary stream was slower than before but she did not strain to void. She felt that she emptied her bladder completely and there was no postmicturition dribbling. She was no longer depressed and was getting out of her house on a regular basis and planned a holiday in Europe.

Further reading

DRIFE, J. O., HILTON, P. and STANTON, S. L. (eds) (1990) *Micturition* (Proceedings of the 21st RCOG Study Group) Springer-Verlag, London

STANTON, S. L. (ed.) (1990) *Clinical Gynaecological Urology*, Churchill Livingstone, London

Case 15

The patient was a 25-year-old factory worker married to a butcher. They were both currently employed. Despite this being their first and a planned pregnancy, the patient had no real recollection of her last menstrual period. The family history was unremarkable. Eight months before, she had presented in the medical department with a 10-month history of intermittent bouts of left iliac fossa pain relieved by passing stool. At times the stools were watery, mucoid and bloodstained. The episodes would last up to a week and occurred at roughly monthly intervals. Her weight had been sustained and the appetite was satisfactory. Colonoscopy with biopsy and barium meal and follow through studies identified inflammatory bowel changes consistent with Crohn's disease. Treatment with mesalazine 400 mgm three times daily was prescribed and on this regimen her symptoms subsided. The patient discontinued the treatment as soon as she thought she was pregnant but there had been no relapse in her symptomatology. She experienced a daily bowel action with a well-formed stool. There had been no rectal bleeding.

On examination she appeared well nourished;she was not clinically anaemic and her general examination was unremarkable apart from tenderness elicited on palpation of the descending colon and deep palpation in the right iliac fossa. She was normotensive, BP 110/70 mmHg. Bimanual examination confirmed an intrauterine pregnancy consistent with a 12-week gestation. The tenderness suggested on abdominal palpation was confirmed during the bimanual examination. Her haemoglobin level was 11.8 g/dl with normal red cell indices. Six weeks later the uterus had grown proportionately and ultrasound examination confirmed a singleton pregnancy with a BPD of 42 mm. The configuration of the fetus appeared normal. Treatment with mesalazine was recommenced. Thereafter her antenatal care progressed without any problems. At 33 weeks the fetus presented by the breech. The breech was not engaged in the pelvis and palpation suggested that the legs were extended. She is now at 37 weeks gestation. The uterine size is equivalent to dates and the breech presentation persists. Weight gain has been consistent throughout the pregnancy.

Questions

What additional investigations and management would you have undertaken during this pregnancy, and why?

Regional enteritis can cause anaemia. This is usually of an iron deficiency pattern but megaloblastic anaemia can occur. Although her initial haemoglobin level was satisfactory it would be prudent to estimate the serum iron, iron binding capacity and ferritin levels on booking if only to confirm basal normal iron status, and then to repeat them at 28, 32 and 36 weeks to detect any deterioration in haemopoiesis. For the same reasons supplementary iron, folate and multivitamins should be supplied. It would seem that this patient's disease is mild and that it has been well controlled on low levels of medication. Nevertheless, it would be advisable to monitor fetal growth by serial ultrasound to exclude intrauterine growth retardation secondary to any malabsorption and because of the association of active disease with intrauterine death. Measurements of the BPD, HC to AC ratio together with an estimation of the maximum liquor pool would suffice at 28, 32 and 36 weeks.

What factors in pregnancy predispose to a breech presentation?

Early gestation	Multiple pregnancy	Uterine abnormality
Fetal abnormality	Polyhydramnios	Oligohydramnios
Cornual insertion of placenta	Placenta praevia	Short cord
Diminished fetal movements	Extended fetal legs	Impaired fetal growth
Contracted pelvis	Maternal consumption of anticonvulsant drugs	Nulliparity
Previous breech		

How would you plan and manage this patient's delivery?

This patient is a young primigravid. Her pregnancy to 37 weeks has been unblemished. There are no associated features such as a history of infertility or bad obstetric history that would colour one's opinion as to the mode of delivery.

It has been calculated that for vaginal delivery the fetal risk with breech presentation, corrected for abnormalities which may have caused the malpresentation, is four times that for cephalic presentation. However, one must weigh against this risk the implications to the mother of the only alternative, a caesarean section. This procedure is associated with a maternal death rate of 0.61 per 1000 operations. It has been estimated that the maternal death rate associated with caesarean section is four times that associated with all vaginal deliveries. Pulmonary embolus, anaesthetic complications, haemorrhage and sepsis are the principal causes of maternal loss from surgery. In addition there is a significant increase in maternal morbidity. Caesarean section in a first pregnancy chequers the patient's subsequent obstetric career. Controlled trials involving cases satisfying strict criteria suggest that term breech fetuses may be delivered safely per vaginum irrespective of parity or the type of breech presentation. The aim of management therefore is to reserve caesarean section for normal babies where vaginal delivery would carry a disproportionate risk or situations where a vaginal delivery is impractical.

In this case, clinically the uterine size is proportional to dates and the fetus does not feel unduly large. Serial ultrasound measurements have been made during the pregnancy and growth has been sustained throughout. The measurements should nevertheless be repeated at 38 weeks to provide an estimate of fetal weight. An estimated fetal weight of 2.5–4.0 kg would be acceptable for attempted vaginal delivery. Beyond these limits the perinatal mortality escalates. On clinical examination the legs are extended and this favourable feature could be confirmed Ultrasound can identify the fetus with an extended neck. Vaginal delivery in such cases carries an additional hazard of transection of the fetal spinal cord and caesarean section would be indicated.

A careful assessment of the pelvic capacity is required. A vaginal examination should be performed paying special attention to the following features: ability/inability to reach the sacral promontory, the curve of the sacrum, the mobility of the coccyx; the length of the sacrospinous ligaments, the prominence of the ischial spines, the convergence (if any) of the pelvic side walls; the width of the subpubic angle, and the intertuberous separation. Ideally the pelvis should manifest the features of the gynaecoid pelvis. If the impression is of an android pelvis with narrowing diameters to the outlet then proportionately larger diameters will be required before contemplating a vaginal delivery. The clinical assessment should be supplemented by an erect lateral pelvimetry. This view of the pelvis will reveal anomalies of the brim such as sacralization of L5, spondylolisthesis, in addition to abnormalities of the sacral curve. Narrowing of the sacrosciatic notch is further evidence of an android pelvis. This information contributes to an appreciation of the shape of the pelvis. In addition, the measurements of the anteroposterior diameters of the brim, midcavity and outlets should each exceed 11.5 cm. Abnormalities of shape contraindicate vaginal delivery as much as reduction in the pelvic diameters unless the latter are capacious.

There have been no pregnancy complications to suggest impaired placental function or which might be construed to threaten placental function. Providing the examinations suggested are satisfactory then this patient would be suitable for a vaginal breech delivery and this is an appropriate time to discuss with the patient the options involved and the significance of the results which lead to the advice given.

If what you say is correct, how do you explain the increasing recourse to caesarean section for the delivery of the breech?

Not all of this increase relates to breech presentation at term. The incidence of breech presentation increases with shorter gestation. As paediatric success with the preterm baby has improved there has been a move to manage complications developing in midpregnancy more aggressively, to deliver these small babies by caesarean section in order to present the paediatrician with a baby in the best possible condition. Caesarean section for breech presentation would seem to be advantageous when the birth-weight is 1000–1500 g, but survival is not affected by mode of delivery when the baby weighs 1500–2500 g. Below 1000 g, although some studies suggest an improved prognosis after operative delivery, other factors operate including the availability of neonatal intensive care, the need frequently to resort to a classical incision or one that encroaches on the upper segment, and the requirement for a high degree of operative skill as the gentle delivery of a fragile baby from a small uterus is not easy.

All breech labours require the highest standards of intrapartum fetal surveillance. This includes continuous fetal heart monitoring either by Doppler or by an electrode applied to the presenting part. In such cases abnormal fetal heart traces will be observed which are not necessarily associated with fetal acidaemia. In a cephalic presentation the true situation can be detected by performing fetal scalp sampling because analysis of fetal scalp blood yields values that reflect the situation in the central vessels. This is not the case with capillary blood obtained from the buttock. Alternative 'norms' for breech capillary samples have been described but these have not been generally adopted and in the event of an abnormal fetal heart trace, most advocate an abdominal delivery.

Operative rates for breech delivery vary considerably not only from country to country but even within countries, between similar institutions and between individuals. The fluctuations are greater than can be accounted for by variations in the case mix. Non-medical determinants play a part. These include the socioeconomic status of the patient and their articulation of their expectations, the influence of increased litigation, the proportion of private practice, convenience for the clinician or unit, and an ever decreasing reservoir of expertise in the vaginal delivery of the breech with the inevitable consequences for teaching and training.

Considerations such as these also make the performance of caesarean section more likely even when the initial decision was to select the patient for a vaginal delivery. Between 18% and 40% of cases selected for vaginal delivery end in caesarean section. Poor progress despite augmentation of labour with Syntocinon is the commonest indication. Emergency caesarean section poses a greater risk to the mother than elective caesarean section especially when executed in the second stage. In one series half the intrapartum caesarean sections took place in the second stage.

Apart from vaginal delivery as a breech and caesarean section are there any other alternatives that might be considered?

Possibly external version to a cephalic presentation and subsequent vaginal delivery. However, this is a nulliparous patient and the uterus is firm and unyielding. It is an extended breech and this too would reduce the chances of success with this manoeuvre at this gestation. The concern is that committed to version excess force might be employed that could result in abruption of the placenta or fetomaternal transfusion, an important consideration in this patient who is Rhesus negative.

Do you recognise any contraindications to external cephalic version?

Any bleeding in pregnancy including first trimester bleeding, hypertensive disorders, previous caesarean section, multiple pregnancy, placenta praevia, an anteriorly situated placenta, fibroids, intrauterine growth retardation, oligohydramnios, and possibly Rhesus negative genotypes.

Are there any hazards?

Abruption of the placenta, fetomaternal transfusion, entanglement of the cord, rupture of the membranes, fetal distress, and the stimulation of preterm labour. Placental localization by ultrasound would identify the anterior placenta which makes version more difficult and increases the risk of abruption and fetomaternal transfusion. If performed in Rhesus negative patients, they require the sampling of maternal blood for a Kleihauer test following version and the administration of 500 units anti-D gamma globulin. In all cases following version a check should be made to exclude vaginal bleeding or the loss of amniotic fluid. The fetal heart rate should be determined before attempted version and afterwards. Bradycardia or irregularity suggest cord entanglement and the option of reversing the version or immediate delivery.

Would you induce labour at term?

No. If before or at term a complication of pregnancy were to supervene that would indicate induction of labour, e.g. pre-eclampsia, then delivery should be by caesarean section. The spontaneous onset of labour should be awaited with regular evaluation of fetal wellbeing by fetal activity recording and cardiotocography. If labour does not supervene by the 12th day past term then delivery should be achieved by caesarean section. This is a somewhat arbitrary demarcation but as the role of prolonged pregnancy and fetal asphyxia is uncertain and the greatest risk to the breech is asphyxia then elective delivery is probably a more defendable alternative to vaginal delivery.

Discussion

Active Crohn's disease is associated with some reduction in fertility usually as a result of oligomenorrhoea or amenorrhoea. When controlled medically or surgically or when in remission fertility is not impaired. Similarly, when the disease is controlled there appears to be no increased risk to the fetus. If however the disease is active during pregnancy, especially at the time of conception or develops during pregnancy, then there is an increased fetal loss, largely through the mechanisms of spontaneous abortion, preterm labour, stillbirth and fetal abnormality. From the quiescent state the relapse rate to active disease in pregnancy is no greater than for the non-pregnant population. In chronic disease with widespread inflammatory changes and adhesions, intestinal obstruction may occur as the disposition of the bowel is altered when the uterus enlarges. In such cases,if conservative measures fail then laparotomy will be necessary. In severe disease and particularly if there is a history of ileal resection or ileocaecal bypass then the patient should receive vitamin B12 throughout pregnancy and the puerperium up to the cessation of lactation. The nutritional state of the mother should be assessed further by estimation of trace elements such as chromium, zinc and copper in the maternal blood. Although rare, colorectal carcinoma is associated with colonic Crohn's disease as well as ulcerative colitis. Usually the inflammatory bowel disease has been present many years but in the event of the patient complaining of rectal bleeding this possibility must be considered in the differential diagnosis.

External cephalic version for the correction of a breech presentation has fallen into disrepute. It was customary to perform this manoeuvre at the time the breech presentation was diagnosed, usually between 32 and 36 weeks. It was demonstrated that version at this time was frequently followed by reversion to the malpresentation and there was always the risk of precipitate intervention in the event of complications such as those listed in the answer above. The fetal loss associated with preterm version was estimated to be as much as 1%. Furthermore, it is possible that following preterm version and before the onset of labour other complications might develop, e.g. APH, pre-eclampsia, IUGR which would demand surgical delivery rendering the version unnecessary. Finally, randomized controlled trials failed to demonstrate any effect of preterm version on the incidence of breech delivery, caesarean section rate or perinatal outcome.

More recently it has been demonstrated that external cephalic version is a feasible proposition at or near term when tocolytics are employed to relax the uterus. The opportunity to correct the presentation will be lost in those cases that go into labour before term, but every opportunity will have been afforded the fetus to undergo spontaneous version before then. The additional complications that may in themselves dictate the mode of delivery will have become manifest and will have been dealt with. Fewer reversions to the malpresentation occur. In the event of any of the complications developing that cause concern when the procedure is carried out preterm, then immediate resort to caesarean section is less problematical when the fetus is known to be mature. Before version an ultrasound examination should be performed to exclude impaired intrauterine growth, and to confirm an adequate volume of amniotic fluid. An anterior placenta may be considered a relative contraindication to version. A cardiotocogram should confirm a reactive trace. General anaesthesia should not be employed because as with preterm external cephalic version there is increased fetal loss. Randomized trials employing this technique have confirmed that it reduces the incidence of breech presentation at birth, and reduces the rate of caesarean section without any increase in fetal loss.

Further reading

BINGHAM, P., HIRD, V. and LILFORD, J. L. (1987) Management of the mature selected breech presentation: an analysis based on the intended method of delivery. *British Journal of Obstetrics and Gynaecology*, **94**, 746–752

COLLEA, J. V., RABIN, S. C., WEGHORST, G. and QUILLIGAN, G. (1978) The randomized management of term breech frank breech presentation: vaginal delivery *versus* cesarean section. *American Journal of Obstetrics and Gynecology*, **131**, 186–195

CROWLEY, P. and HAWKINS, D. F. (1980) Premature breech delivery: the caesarean section debate. *Journal of Obstetrics and Gynaecology*, **1**, 2–6

GIMOUSKY, M. L., PETRIE, R. H. and RODD, N. D. (1980) Neonatal performance of the selected term vaginal delivery. *Obstetrics and Gynecology*, **109**, 418–120

HOFMEYER, G. J. (1983) Effect of external cephalic version in late pregnancy on breech presentation and caesarean section rate: a controlled trial. *British Journal of Obstetrics and Gynaecology*, **90**, 392–399

MILLER, J. P. (1986) Inflammatory bowel disease in pregnancy: a review. *Journal of the Royal Society of Medicine*, **79**, 221–225

WEAVER, J. (1980) Breech delivery: obstetric outcome. In *Outcomes of Obstetric Intervention in Britain*. Proceedings of a scientific meeting of the Royal College of Obstetricians and Gynaecologists (29 May 1986) (eds R. W. Beard and D. B. Paintin) pp.47–59

Case 16

The anxious 62-year-old widow of a shipyard worker was referred to the gynaecological clinic by the hospital physician. She was known to have extensive sigmoid diverticular disease which exacerbated from time to time with rectal bleeding. These symptoms had been controlled with bran supplements. She had suffered from chronic obstructive airways disease for most of her adult life and this was controlled by salbutamol and becotide inhalation. She had always had a 'weight problem'. At 36 years of age she had suffered from menorrhagia and she requested a sterilization procedure. She had six children by this time all delivered normally. Her first pregnancy had been at the age of 16 years. The patient underwent an operative procedure and was told that she had had a hysterectomy. However, her GP's first letter to the physicians referred to a subtotal hysterectomy and left salpingo-oophorectomy. Following this surgery she had never had a cervical smear. She had complained to her medical advisers of bleeding per vaginum on two occasions. The first had been 8 months before referral to the gynaecological clinic when she experienced a scanty slightly offensive dark red loss over 3 days. A speculum and vaginal examination at that time revealed no abnormalities and she was reassured that all was well. The second episode had been a month before being seen in the clinic when there was a bright red loss sufficient to stain her underclothing but which resolved within 24 h. There was no pain. She was certain that the loss did not originate from the rectum. She also complained of vague chest pain associated with occasional palpitations but no swelling of the ankles. She had episodes of paroxysmal nocturnal dyspnoea and orthopnoea.

On examination the patient was small (157.5 cm) and very obese weighing 84.5 kg. Her BP was 170/110 mmHg and her pulse 90 beats/min. There was no peripheral oedema or signs of congestive heart failure. Chest expansion was poor;the breath sounds were normal but with prolonged expiration consistent with mild bronchospasm. The abdomen was obese with a prominent 'apron'; there was a midline subumbilical scar from the subtotal hysterectomy. The external genitalia were normal. The perineum was very deficient, however, and the introitus gaped to reveal the posterior vaginal wall, changes in keeping with her high parity. The vagina was lax but there was no overt vaginal wall prolapse. There was no vaginitis and scraping the vaginal wall failed to produce any petechiae or bleeding. The cervix looked entirely normal and there was no descent on straining. Bimanual examination was difficult because of her obesity but the vault of the vagina was mobile and supple and there were no masses palpable in the pelvis. A rectal examination and proctoscopy were normal.

How would you manage this case?

There is a clear history of postmenopausal bleeding. The examination of the patient identifies no local lesion to explain the loss. The patient has had a subtotal hysterectomy in the past. The cervix appears normal but it could harbour some pathology responsible for the bleeding. If the level of transection did not remove all the endometrium then sufficient might remain to be the focus of malignant change or be activated by hormonal activity from the remaining ovary. I would request a cervical smear including endocervical brush cytology, an ultrasound examination of the pelvis, and the serum oestradiol and gonadotrophin levels.

This patient is 62 years old, what kind of ovarian activity do you mean?

There is always the possibility of an oestrogen secreting tumour such as a granulosa cell tumour or thecoma. These can be small and undetected on routine examination and this lady is particularly obese. Even non-endocrine tumours of the ovary can result in the secretion of oestrogen, presumably by evoking a stromal response within the ovary.

The cervical smear taken with an Ayre's spatula has been reported as negative. Superficial and intermediate squames, endocervical cells and a number of polymorphs were seen. An ultrasound examination of the pelvis was difficult but no ovarian enlargement was identified. The hormonal assays you requested are consistent with the menopause. What do you want to do?

There have been two episodes of bleeding. The patient is a reliable witness and distinguishes clearly the bleeding on this occasion from the bleeding she associates with her diverticular disease and proctoscopy was normal. The concern must remain despite the negative cytology that pathology resides within the cervical stump. I would want to admit this patient for examination under anaesthesia and excision of the cervical stump.

Are there any precautions that you would take?

She has a history of chronic obstructive airways disease and ill-defined chest pain. A chest X-ray, ECG, and full blood count would be necessary preliminaries before discussing with her physician and the anaesthetist the optimum mode of anaesthesia. Surgery under an epidural anaesthetic might be advisable. She is obese and at greater risk for deep vein thrombosis and pulmonary embolism. Prophylactic anticoagulation with s.c. heparin, the use of anti-embolic stockings and early mobilization after her operation are all advisable in her case.

What would be your regimen for DVT prophylaxis?

Calcium heparin 5 000 units s.c. 2 h before surgery and then every 8 h for 7 days.

Why do you think this patient had a subtotal hysterectomy?

It is hard to say. The patient was told that she had had a hysterectomy, and although no mention was made of surgical difficulty at the time, she has always been obese and there may have been difficulty with access. The operation was performed some years ago when it was a more popular procedure. The operation is easier and quicker to perform than the total hysterectomy. It involves less risk to the bladder, ureters and rectum. If access is limited or the anaesthetic causes concern then recourse to this procedure can be understood.

It was felt that the subtotal operation preserved the length of the vagina for coitus and did not leave a scar at the vault to cause dyspareunia. In fact, a total hysterectomy does not significantly shorten the vagina and coitus itself by stretching the tissues solves the problem if any.

Some surgeons preferred to retain the cervix if possible to sustain vaginal lubrication from the endocervical secretions. In fact, lubrication at coitus which is the usual concern, is mediated by the activity of Bartholin's glands. Concerns that the cervix is essential for the achievement of an orgasm is ill-founded in fact.

It was argued that by leaving the cervix with its attached transverse cervical and uterosacral ligamentary attachments intact that the vault would remain supported. However, when these very supports slacken after the menopause the cervix can form the apex of a vault prolapse.

Are there any actual disadvantages to this procedure?

In the event of any pelvic collection developing after surgery drainage is more difficult if the cervix is intact. The stump can become the site of infection producing chronic cervicitis, discharge and dyspareunia. If the removal of the uterine isthmus has not been complete then menstrual or ovulatory bleeding may continue. Fibroids have been described growing from the cervical stump. Finally, there is always the risk of dysplasia or frank malignancy developing in the cervical remnant at a later date.

Is there any place for the subtotal operation in modern gynaecological surgery?

If the misconceptions about the benefit of the procedure are excluded then the indications for the operation must be infrequent. There is a school which interprets the use of the subtotal hysterectomy as the reflection of an inadequate surgical technique. This is an extreme view, and like all extreme views, potentially dangerous if it results in a surgeon pursuing an inappropriate operation for the sake of dogma. There may be situations where the surgeon feels that because of pathology in the pouch of Douglas, such as fibrosis secondary to pelvic inflammatory disease or distortion of the anatomy because of burnt out endometriosis, the subtotal operation offers the solution to the patient's symptoms with the minimal risk to adjacent structures.

With modern anaesthesia and relaxants limited access to the pelvis is seldom a problem. The occasions where the operation may be required will be few but the technique should not be discarded from the repertoire.

Outcome

The patient underwent a thorough pelvic examination and removal of the cervical stump under an epidural anaesthetic. Her recovery was complete.

The cervical stump measured 2.0 × 3.0 × 1.5 cm and was grossly normal. Histological examination revealed a heavy inflammatory infiltrate suggestive of chronic cervicitis. The epithelium adjacent to the squamocolumnar junction in the cervical canal showed a single area of severe dysplasia consistent with a diagnosis of carcinoma *in situ* (CIN III). The lesion had been completely excised.

Discussion

The case highlights the need to communicate adequately with the patient. She was unaware that the cervix had been left *in situ*. No directions had been given to her or to her GP that she would require regular cervical cytology screening like any other woman. There is a danger when patients are discharged from hospital before the histological report on the operative specimen is available that the standard discharge letter, referring to a hysterectomy having been successfully completed, might be taken to imply that there was no cause for further concern. The GP should be informed of the precise histological state of the cervix in the operative specimen. Patients who have a hysterectomy for carcinoma *in situ*, or in whose operative specimen carcinoma *in situ* is discovered unexpectedly, require cytological follow-up with vault smears, probably annually. It follows that after a routine hysterectomy for benign indications a purposeful histological examination of the cervix is desirable to exclude preinvasive disease. Because in most units only token blocks of tissue are examined histologically from the cervix after a hysterectomy for benign pathology there is a good argument to advise vault smears from such patients at the routine recall intervals.

It is estimated that there is a 0.5–1.0% risk of carcinoma of the cervix developing within 10 years of a subtotal hysterectomy. The carcinoma may have been present but unsuspected at the time of the initial surgery. More usually it originates *de novo* in the cervical stump and malignant change appears to be more common when the operation has been performed for pelvic infection. Such cases usually reflect a degree of sexual activity and it may be this dimension that is responsible for an apparent, rather than a real, association as cervical precancer has been attributed directly to sexual activity.

The cancer, once initiated, progresses like any cancer of the cervix but because the bladder, rectum and peritoneal cavity are immediately adjacent to the stump infiltration of these organs takes place more rapidly. The anatomy is distorted and radical surgery may be more difficult than usual. Furthermore, the uterus is not available as a location for a radiotherapy source in advanced disease. Stump carcinoma therefore enjoys a bad reputation and 5-year survival rates vary between 30% and 60%.

This patient had a negative cervical smear immediately before surgery. In the menopause the squamocolumnar junction usually lies within the endocervical canal. The negative result represents a sampling error even though some endocervical cells were reported in the smear. In a patient of this age, certainly with symptoms, it might have been wiser to use a better shaped spatula, e.g. an Aylesbury spatula and/or an endocervical brush cytology specimen.

Comment

The examination here, as is usually the case, is based on the evaluation of the history and a reasoned programme of management based on the candidates appraisal of the patient both from the medical and the gynaecological points of view. The general examination in this case is as significant as the gynaecological examination. The subject matter covered is not to be found in profound review literature. The issues discussed are part of the general knowledge of the candidate acquired during his day to day training. The candidate should be capable of demonstrating the use of the proctoscope.

Case 17

The patient was a 28-year-old bank clerk in her third pregnancy. She was married to an accountant. Her past medical history had been uneventful and the family and social histories unexceptional. She booked into the antenatal clinic at a district general hospital on 31 March. Her last menstrual period had been on the 12 January. She reported a regular menstrual cycle, 5/35–40, and had used barrier methods for contraception since the birth of her last child a year ago.

Her first pregnancy had ended with a spontaneous abortion at 10 weeks gestation. The second pregnancy a year later progressed normally to 33 weeks gestation when spontaneous labour supervened and she was delivered of a live female infant weighing 1580 g, which thrived. There was no history of urinary tract infection, premature rupture of the membranes or haemorrhage. The labour was relatively silent in its onset, the patient being 'well on' when admitted. She understood that 'there was something funny with the womb' but had no memory of any investigations to confirm this diagnosis.

In the current pregnancy she had felt well since the onset. An ultrasound examination at the booking visit confirmed a single gestation sac containing a fetus with a CRL of 41 mm. On examination she was reassured that she was indeed pregnant and that the cervix was tightly closed.

She was referred for shared antenatal care until 34 weeks gestation. On 18 August the patient presented as an emergency at her base hospital 22 miles from the teaching unit. At 08.00 hours she had experienced abdominal discomfort which by 10.00 hours had become recognizable as uterine contractions every 10 min. There had been no bleeding or vaginal loss to suggest the leakage of amniotic fluid. On admission to the district hospital an examination confirmed that the cervix was fully effaced and 3 cm dilated. The membranes were intact and bulging through the os. The uterus felt smallish for dates. The fetus presented by the head. An infusion of ritodrine was started, and after discussing the situation with the paediatrician and obstetrician in the regional referral centre, a transfer of the mother to the centre was organized.

On arrival at 14.00 hours the uterine activity had ceased. The patient was receiving ritodrine 12 mgm/h by infusion. The infusion was tailed off and oral therapy substituted. The patient is currently taking 10 mgm ritodrine every 6 h. Since admission there has been no recurrence of the uterine activity. On dates she is now 33 weeks pregnant.

Questions

What are the essential points of the history so far?

This is a patient at increased risk for preterm labour. She has had a previous preterm delivery and there is a suggestion of a uterine abnormality. The validity of this is unsure as it would seem that the patient has not had an hysterosalpingogram between pregnancies and no comment was made as to an abnormality of the uterus at the time of her recent ultrasound examination.

There would seem to be a doubt as to the gestation of the pregnancy. She has a long cycle and from the values given for her early ultrasound the gestational age is probably 2 weeks behind the dates calculated from the LMP.

The changes described in the cervix would confirm that she had been in labour and that the situation had been controlled by the administration of betamimetics.

What do you mean by the term preterm labour?

The spontaneous onset of labour 21 days or more before term.

What factors are associated with the onset of preterm labour?

Poor social circumstances	Age $<$20 years or $>$35 years	Small stature
Smoking	Increasing parity	Previous perinatal loss
Previous preterm labour	Previous antepartum haemorrhage	Cervical trauma
Previous therapeutic abortion	Previous spontaneous abortion	Polyhydramnios
Maternal infection or pyrexia	Bleeding in pregnancy	Multiple pregnancy
Congenital malformation	Uterine malformation	Pre-eclampsia
Intrauterine death	Iatrogenic interference	Premature rupture of the membranes

This patient has been the subject of an intrauterine transfer because of preterm labour. What requirements do you think need to be satisfied before planning a transfer, and how would you organize it?

The reason for considering a transfer is that the facilities available at the base hospital are insufficient to manage adequately a baby or babies delivered at that gestation. There can be no absolute rule to dictate the gestation at which transfer must take place. In a unit with limited facilities, the transfer of women in labour up to 36 completed weeks would be reasonable. If the unit has designated special care cots, then only mothers in labour before 31 weeks might be transferred. The prospect of a delivery before this time would indicate a need for neonatal intensive care and transfer to a regional unit.

A necessary prerequisite to any request for intrauterine transfer is a careful reappraisal of the gestational age based on such data as is available. Gestational age in these problem pregnancies is a better determinant of infant outcome than estimates of fetal weight.

Every effort must be made to avoid transfer under emergency conditions. If preterm labour is suspected, then early transfer is advisable, even if subsequently definitive labour does not establish. If the reason to transfer the patient is because of a deteriorating maternal or fetal condition then it is unreasonable to have the patient in hospital for days only to request transfer when the situation has become critical.

In the event of preterm labour the transfer must be realistic. The distance between the units and the local geography will dictate the travelling time. These factors need to be balanced against the cervical dilatation, the dynamics of labour at the proposed time of transfer and the patient's performance in any earlier pregnancy.

Whatever the concern may be for the fetus, the wisdom of any transfer is dictated by any risk to the mother. If the travelling time is long then the transfer of a mother with a significant APH or severe pre-eclampsia may be inappropriate. Because of these complex variables, negotiations to transfer such patients should be made only between senior staff who have personally assessed the situation in the base hospital, and the consultant obstetrician and paediatrician at the regional centre.

Depending on the exact circumstances, the transfer may be accomplished under the cover of tocolytic therapy and possibly the administration of steroids to promote pulmonary maturation.

The transfer of the patient requires a suitably equipped

ambulance. The patient should be accompanied by a doctor and midwife to undertake delivery should it be necessary and to supervise medication during transfer. An intravenous infusion is a wise precaution if not already *in situ*.

If there is any doubt as to the prudence of a transfer then it should not be undertaken. An alternative is to summons a paediatric flying squad to attend a preterm delivery or to collect the baby after delivery if its condition warrants it. The evidence is however, that the prognosis for the preterm baby is enhanced by antenatal referral to a greater degree than for neonatal transfer.

Such transfers represent an enormous dislocation for the mother and her family. The possibility of transfer should be discussed with the parents at the earliest opportunity rather than confronting them with an apparent fait accompli in addition to all the other anxieties they will have at this time.

What agents are you aware of that might be used to suppress preterm labour?

Betamimetic drugs	Prostaglandin synthesis inhibitors	Calcium antagonists
Ethanol infusion	Magnesium sulphate	Progesterone
Diazoxide	Oxytocin analogues	

With which of these preparations have you had any personal experience?

Ritodrine, a betamimetic.

How would you use this? Why do you choose it and are there any side-effects?

Trials have established that betamimetics are successful in delaying labour and reducing the incidence of preterm birth when compared with controls. Alone, they do not influence the perinatal mortality or morbidity. Their main uses are to delay labour so that the administration of corticosteroids may have an effect in promoting pulmonary maturity and to enable the transfer of a mother to a centre with neonatal intensive care facilities. Ritodrine is an agent that has,in controlled trials against placebo, been shown to achieve these effects.

A solution is prepared of 100 mgm ritodrine in 500 ml of 5% dextrose. An intravenous infusion is commenced at an initial rate of 15 ml/h increasing every 10 min by 15 ml/h until contractions cease or an infusion rate of 105 ml/h maximum is reached. The maternal heart rate and blood pressure should be recorded every 10 min and the patient asked about possible side-effects.

Should the maternal pulse rate exceed 140 beats/min, palpitations or other severe side-effects occur then the infusion rate should be halved; if any symptoms do not subside within 10 min the infusion should be stopped. When the uterine contractions have been stopped, the effective infusion rate should be continued for a further hour. The rate is then halved and discontinued after a further 6 h. Two hours before the cessation of intravenous therapy oral therapy is commenced. Ritodrine 10 mgm is prescribed 4-hourly for 48 h and thereafter 6-hourly.

Although it is claimed that ritodrine exerts a predominant effect on beta-2 receptors there is still some stimulation of beta-1 receptors and the patients may complain of palpitations, nausea, vomiting, tremor, headache, and restlessness. Tocolysis is unlikely to be achieved if the maternal heart rate is below 100 beats/min. An increase in pulse pressure is observed. There will be an increase in cardiac output over and above that from the pregnancy. The problem will be more pronounced in a multiple pregnancy and patients with hyperthyroidism. In patients with undiagnosed heart conditions severe cardiac compromise can result. Signs of myocardial ischaemia may be unmasked during therapy. An ECG before treatment would seem to be a wise precaution.

Pulmonary oedema may result from fluid overload, usually when correcting maternal hypotension, in association with those betamimetics with a greater beta-1 activity, e.g. isoxsuprine. Betamimetics also may have an antidiuretic effect, at least in the first 48 h of treatment and overload is more likely if dilute infusions are used. Dextrose would seem to pose less of a problem than saline. A careful fluid balance record is obligatory. The complication has been recorded most frequently in multiple pregnancies. Overload should be suspected if the patient develops tachypnoea and feels short of breath especially when supine. Tachycardia is the rule usually in excess of 130 beats/min. Despite the hyperventilation P_{O_2} will be reduced. If pulmonary oedema is suspected then the betamimetic should be stopped and oxygen administered. Diuretics may be necessary and in severe cases the condition may demand artificial ventilation.

Betamimetics induce hyperglycaemia, hyperinsulinaemia and lipolysis. The effects are accentuated in diabetic women and can precipitate severe ketoacidosis. These metabolic effects may be made worse by the giving of corticosteroids to promote fetal pulmonary maturity. The betamimetics cross the placenta and induce metabolic effects in the fetus to produce hypoglycaemia and hyperinsulinaemia after birth. There should be frequent assessment of the fetal blood sugar after birth following the use of tocolytics in labour.

To minimize the side-effects of betamimetics, calcium antagonists and beta-1 receptor blockers have been used in combination with them. There is no evidence that the concurrent use of such drugs protects the mother against the complications of betamimetic therapy.

Because of the effects of betamimetics on the maternal circulation the interpretation of physical signs in association with vaginal bleeding becomes difficult. The hyperdynamic circulation might aggravate a tendency to haemorrhage. The drugs are best avoided where preterm labour is associated with vaginal bleeding.

How would you deliver this patient if labour were to supervene now?

Before undertaking the delivery of this patient I would require a detailed ultrasound examination of the fetus. The only ultrasound reported was performed in early pregnancy at 12 weeks gestation. A scan now would positively exclude a multiple pregnancy and identify serious fetal abnormalities and possible growth retardation; all associated with preterm labour, and which would influence the decision as to the mode of delivery. Ultrasound would also confirm the presentation of the fetus and its attitude. There is no maternal complication to dictate the mode of delivery, e.g. fulminating pre-eclampsia. There have been no other complications of pregnancy. I would allow labour to progress normally anticipating a vaginal delivery. An epidural anaesthetic would avoid the use of narcotics that might inhibit breathing at birth. I would monitor the fetus electronically undertaking fetal scalp sampling if the trace caused concern and intervening surgically if fetal acidaemia were confirmed. There is no evidence that prophylactic forceps delivery improves the outcome for the preterm fetus, rather the reverse. I would perform an episiotomy sufficient only to achieve a controlled delivery of the fetal head. The delivery should be conducted by an experienced attendant. An experienced neonatologist should be present at the delivery should resuscitation be necessary. Particular attention should be paid to the protection of the fetus from cold after delivery.

Discussion

The administration of corticosteroids to the mother in preterm labour to promote fetal lung maturation has not been universally accepted. Initially there was concern from some animal studies, that organ differentiation was being promoted at the expense of cell division and organ growth, and this effect included the fetal brain. The doses used in these experiments were significantly larger than those used in human pregnancy. The usual doses prescribed are 24 mgm betamethasone, 24 mgm dexamethasone or 2 g hydrocortisone. Follow-up studies on babies subjected to glucocorticoids in association with preterm labour have to date shown no impairment of intellectual or functional capacity.

There can be no reasonable doubt that glucocorticoids do reduce the incidence of idiopathic respiratory distress syndrome of the newborn, periventricular haemorrhage and necrotizing enterocolitis. Furthermore, these effects are maximal when delivery takes place more than 24 h and less than 7 days after the giving of the drug. The effect is irrespective of the sex of the fetus. It is possible that the effect is less pronounced in association with multiple pregnancy. Even outside these time limits the giving of these drugs produces benefit. One use of betamimetics is to allow this therapeutic window to be realized in the event of preterm labour. Care must be taken in combining therapies. Cases have been reported of maternal pulmonary oedema when corticosteroids have been given in association with betamimetics and magnesium sulphate. There may be an increase in the risk of maternal infection. Diabetes, hypertensive disease, IUGR, are each conditions which dictate early delivery and which would seem ideal to be covered by corticosteroids to promote fetal lung maturation.

In the diabetic, fetal hyperinsulinism may cause cortisol resistance in the fetal lung, thus reducing its effect. Corticosteroids may induce a loss of diabetic control, risking ketoacidosis which increases perinatal loss. When corticosteroids are administered until delivery (24–48 h) the use of a dextrose/potassium/insulin infusion monitored by the maternal blood sugar estimations would be the safest method of judging the maternal insulin requirement.

Early reports suggested that in hypertensive disease fetal loss was increased further by the giving of corticosteroids. In part, this effect was observed because the treatment group contained a disproportionate number of severe pre-eclamptics. An increase in perinatal loss has not been seen in more recent trials. If the maternal condition is worsening rapidly then delay to await the effects of corticosteroids is not justified.

The advantage of corticosteroids in the management of planned delivery for IUGR or Rhesus disease is more obscure as they themselves may alter the dynamics of surfactant production in the fetus *in utero*.

Comment

The initial questions in this case could be asked before the patient's examination has been undertaken in front of the examiners. The history alone triggers certain questions and the examiner wishes to assess the response. The examiner led with the simplest of questions. There was no trick. The next question was a straightforward enquiry into book knowledge. The candidate, hopefully now relaxed, was asked to reveal his practical experience and the lessons he has learned. The pattern of questioning was then repeated. The examiner was interested in learning not only the candidate's response to given situations but also his awareness of the limitations of his options and the risks of his treatment. The theoretical questions opened many options for the examiner who might have chosen to test the candidate further on knowledge beyond his practical experience, e.g. the possible role of calcium antagonists in the management of preterm labour. Finally, the questioning led into a controversial area where the opinion of the candidate was specifically requested.

Outcome

A detailed ultrasound examination at 33 weeks confirmed a normal singleton fetus but the fetal measurements suggested that the gestational age was less than the 'dates' indicated. The fetus was symmetrically grown and the estimated fetal weight was 1450 g. The placenta was normally situated and there was no suggestion of retroplacental bleeding. There was a second episode of preterm labour at this time which rapidly subsided on tocolytic therapy. Corticosteroids were not given. At 36 weeks by dates the patient was returned to her base hospital. She went into definitive labour at 38 weeks gestation and was delivered of a healthy female infant weighing 2100 g. The paediatric estimation of the fetal age was 36 weeks.

Further reading

HEINONEN, K., HAKULINEN, A. and JOKELA, V. (1988) Survival of the smallest. Time trends and determinents of mortality in a very preterm population during the 1980s. *Lancet*, **2**, 204–207

CROWLEY, P., CHALMERS, I. and KIERSE, M. J. N. C. (1990) The effects of corticosteroid administration before preterm delivery:an overview of the evidence from controlled trials. *British Journal of Obstetrics and Gynaecology*, **97**, 11–25

O'DRISCOLL, K., MEAGHER, D., MacDONALD, D. and GEOGHEGAN, F. (1981) Traumatic intracranial haemorrhage in firstborn infants and delivery with obstetric forceps. *British Journal of Obstetrics and Gynaecology*, **88**, 577–581

PANETH, N., KIELY, J. L., WALLENSTEIN, S. and SUSSER, M. (1987) The choice of place of delivery. Effect of hospital level in all singleton births 'in New York City. *American Journal of Disease of the Child*, **141**, 60–64

Case 18

A 69-year-old widow who had worked for many years as a waitress in the hospital canteen was admitted to the ward as an emergency at the request of her GP. She had commenced bleeding per vaginum 3 days before and the loss had been heavy for the 2 days before admission. The loss had resembled menstrual blood and was not offensive. Closer questioning confirmed that she had experienced intermittent blood loss, never very heavy, for 3 months. There had never been any pain. She could not remember precisely when she had had the menopause but felt that it had been at about 45 years of age. Her menarche had been earlier than some of her friends, she thought at the age of 11 or 12 years. She had never had any problems with the menses. Although she and her husband had been married for 30 years there were no children. They had not sought help from this point of view believing that 'if they were to have come they would have done so'. Her husband had died 19 years ago. There had never been any other partner. She had always enjoyed the best of health and was a non-smoker. She knew of no allergies or sensitivities to drugs. She was taking no medication.

On examination she was a healthy slim woman. She was not anaemic. Her BP was 170/90 mmHg. Her general examination was satisfactory except for prominent varicosities in the long saphenous system of both lower limbs. She attributed these to her occupation observing that they had started to develop when she was young and were certainly not of recent origin. Palpation of the abdomen was normal although a soft liver edge could be palpated two fingers breadth below the right costal margin. There was no ascites.

On pelvic examination the external genitalia looked normal. A speculum was passed easily and a normal-looking cervix visualized with dark blood passing through the os from above. On bimanual examination the uterus was deviated to the right. It was enlarged to the size of a 10-week pregnancy and was irregular in outline. The consistency of the uterus was variable being in some parts firm and elsewhere soft. On the left side a firm mass was palpable approximately 6 cm in diameter. This mass was not clearly demarcated from the uterus and moved with it on displacement. Rectal examination confirmed the findings.

The patient was admitted forthwith and the following day a D and C was performed. The procedure was well tolerated. She was readmitted 2 weeks later, for further surgery.

Questions

On the history given to you by the patient what are your conclusions?

The patient presented with significant postmenopausal bleeding. On examination the uterus is enlarged and irregular. The clinical picture suggests a fibroid uterus. Curettage, however, has presumably identified some pathology because she has been admitted for further surgery, probably a hysterectomy. The patient was instructed not to divulge the nature of the operation. If this is the case then the possibility of an endometrial carcinoma is the first consideration. The combination of an enlarged uterus, postmenopausal bleeding and pathology on curettage would fit this picture.

Is there another possibility? Consider your findings early in your pelvic examination, bearing in mind her circumstances.

There was little genital atrophy. Instrumentation of the vagina was easier than expected from the history of nulliparity and no sexual activity. The vagina was moist. There was no senile vaginitis. The picture was of a well-oestrogenized lower genital tract. Bimanual examination failed to demonstrate a separate adnexal mass but nevertheless the possibility of an ovarian oestrogen-secreting tumour comes to mind, as in giving the history she excluded the possibility of taking extraneous oestrogen.

What then were the likely findings on curettage?

The presence of an oestrogen-secreting tumour would not exclude the finding of endometrial carcinoma. The unopposed oestrogen can induce malignant change in the endometrium. Other changes possible are cystic glandular hyperplasia or atypical glandular hyperplasia.

What oestrogen-secreting tumours do you know of? Can there be any other explanation for her hyperoestronism?

The granulosa cell tumour is the commonest ovarian tumour to produce clinically obvious manifestations, although a quarter of them have no such effects. Theca cell tumours can simulate the clinical picture and more rarely Sertoli–Leydig tumours (androblastomas) and lipoid cell tumours of the ovary. Especially in the postmenopausal age group a variety of neoplasms can induce a functional response in the ovarian stroma. Common epithelial tumours including mucinous, endometrioid, Brenner and metastatic carcinoma can evoke this response and present with postmenopausal bleeding.

She in fact had a fractional curettage, the cervical canal was normal and fragments of healthy columnar epithelium were obtained. The uterine cavity was distorted by fibroids, such endometrium as was obtained was reported as showing cystic glandular hyperplasia. What would be your own management now?

Hyperoestronism is present. It would be academic and unnecessary to seek further proof with estimations of serum gonadotrophins and oestradiol. There is an association between endometrial hyperplasia and diabetes mellitus. A glucose tolerance test should be performed. An ultrasound examination of the pelvis might clarify the situation in the pelvis before surgery and possibly identify an ovarian tumour, but the need to proceed to laparotomy, total hysterectomy and bilateral oophorectomy remains. If there is an ovarian tumour then it may be malignant and the surgery is justified on those grounds alone. Even so the uterus is enlarged by fibroids and the cavity was distorted at curettage hence a focus of endometrial carcinoma within the uterus cannot be excluded. A CT scan of the abdomen however might be of value. The patient offers no symptomatology to suggest other intra-abdominal disease but secondary deposits in the ovary as explained can reproduce this clinical picture. This is particularly the case when the primary lies within the gastrointestinal tract. The examination would also reveal any involvement of the para-aortic glands. A chest X-ray should also be taken. The approach at surgery should be as for an ovarian tumour. Any ascitic fluid should be sent for cytological examination. In the absence of free fluid, peritoneal washings should be taken. There should be a scrupulous inspection of the abdominal cavity to identify any secondary dissemination. It is vital that the staging of any ovarian tumour be as detailed as possible.

Accepting that any malignancy or innocent neoplasms in the ovaries, tubes, corpus, cervix, vagina and vulva can present as postmenopausal bleeding, what other causes of postmenopausal haemorrhage occur?

The most important is the use of extraneous oestrogen therapy. Not uncommon is the mistaken use of unopposed oestrogen for relatively mild symptoms that are assumed to be 'menopausal', although sometimes the menopause may have occurred years before. 'Short trials' of oestrogen without progesterone are unacceptable. Infection can produce bleeding, especially with *Trichomonas* or *Candida*. Senile vaginitis is a common cause of postmenopausal bleeding particularly after infrequent intercourse. Persistent ulceration from tuberculous endometritis can produce a bloodstained discharge. Pyometra and haematometra are more obvious. Trauma to the vagina is possible. Unless checked frequently ring pessaries can produce vaginal ulceration and bleeding. Decubital ulceration on the prolapsed cervix is another possibility. The patient may have developed a bleeding diathesis caused by capillary or haematological disease. The site of bleeding also may have been mistaken by the patient, the problem lying within the urethra, bladder or rectum. Urethral caruncles, papilloma or carcinoma of the bladder, haemorrhoids, fissures and carcinoma of the rectum are possibilities.

Discussion

Postmenopausal bleeding is a symptom which requires immediate investigation. An arbitrary interval of 12 months after the last recorded period is sometimes designated for the diagnosis. However, the pathology may be present already in the climacteric and the distinction between pre- and postmenopausal bleeding will not be recognized. If there is any doubt in the mind of the gynaecologist then investigation is mandatory. It is also advisable to investigate menstruation apparently continuing after 55 years of age to exclude endometrial atypia.

Even if an apparent explanation is discovered, e.g. senile vaginitis, a cervical polyp or extraneous oestrogen and the patient has reported but a single loss, examination under anaesthesia and ideally hysteroscopy and diagnostic curettage is essential. The presence of such factors do not in themselves exclude the possibility of endometrial carcinoma. If then no cause is found within the genital tract and haemorrhage recurs then the urinary and lower gastrointestinal tract should be investigated including sigmoidoscopy and cystoscopy. If the problem persists then laparotomy and hysterectomy will have to be considered as the only means of identifying a small tumour of the ovary or tube or an early carcinoma of the endometrium.

Granulosa cell tumours account for only 1.5% of all ovarian tumours and 6% of ovarian cancers. Two-thirds present after the menopause usually with postmenopausal bleeding. The tumour is usually palpable on pelvic examination (88% of cases). The granulosa cell tumour is prone to rupture and may present as an acute abdomen with a haemoperitoneum. It is unilateral in 95% of cases and usually Stage 1. The prognosis is excellent in such cases with survival at 10 years ranging from 86% to 96%. Two features worsen the prognosis:rupture of the tumour and its initial size. Tumours $\leq$5 cm in diameter have a particularly good prognosis. For these reasons a small Stage Ia tumour in a young patient who wishes to preserve her reproductive capacity can be treated by unilateral oophorectomy. High stage tumours and recurrent tumours may respond well to radiation therapy.

Malignant change in the endometrium is found in approximately 5% of all women with granulosa cell tumours. When endometrial malignancy does supervene it is almost inevitably well differentiated and of low grade.

Granulosa cell tumours are not inevitably hormonally active. In a quarter of cases they are inert. Neither are they necessarily oestrogenic in their manifestation, rarely they can be androgenic. Immunocytochemical studies confirm that granulosa cells from granulosa cell tumours characteristically contained oestradiol but also testosterone and progesterone. Likewise, androblastomas uniformly contain testosterone and oestradiol and occasionally progesterone. Classification of these hormones in the past has been based upon their morphological features or their endocrine manifestations. Both classifications are compromised by the fact that these neoplasms present with variable hormone profiles and frequently complex inter-related histological patterns. Recognition of the diverse capacity for steroid synthesis by these cells explains the variable and sometimes paradoxical hormonal expression that such tumours display.

Outcome

At laparotomy the uterus was enlarged to 10-week size by multiple fibroids. The left ovary was replaced by a solid tumour 5.5 cm in diameter. The capsule was intact. The right ovary was small and fibrotic. There was no ascites and a comprehensive exploration of the abdominal contents demonstrated no pathology. A total hysterectomy and bilateral salpingo-oophorectomy was performed. The histology was reported as follows:

The uterus is enlarged by multiple small fibroids. The endometrium measures up to 0.8 cm thick. The myometrium is thickened measuring up to 2.5 cm. The left ovary is replaced by a well-encapsulated tumour nodule measuring 5.0 × 3.5 × 4.5 cm, grey- white in colour. There is no normal ovarian tissue present. The left ovarian tumour is a granulosa cell tumour showing a predominantly microfollicular type of pattern with the formation of numerous Call Exner bodies. Occasional mitoses are seen but fat is not demonstrated. The endometrium shows cystic glandular hyperplasia with no atypia. The right ovary is unremarkable.

When seen for review she was well and symptom free. She did not complain of flushes or other such symptoms. She remains well under permanent review.

Comment

Postmenopausal bleeding is a problem of such importance that the candidate cannot afford to slip up. If nowhere else, mention must be made during the examination of an intention to carry out a rectal examination and possibly a proctoscopy. It is a useful tip to look specifically for signs of oestrogenization of the vulva and vagina in a case of postmenopausal bleeding.

Further reading

FOX, H., AGRAWAL, K. and LANGLEY, F. A. (1975) A clinicopathological study of 92 cases of granulosa cell tumour of the ovary with special reference to the factors influencing prognosis. *Cancer*, **35**, 231–241

Case 19

The patient was referred to a regional centre because of a known history of Rhesus isoimmunization. Her LMP was on the 20 July and she presented in the antenatal clinic on the 6th October at 11 weeks gestation. The patient was well and normotensive. An ultrasound examination confirmed a singleton pregnancy. The fetus had a crown rump length of 40 mm.

In 1984 the patient had been delivered at her district hospital of a live female infant weighing 3200 g. She was known to be A Rhesus negative but routine antibody screening at 28 and 34 weeks yielded no antibody. The pregnancy was entirely uneventful. The cord blood was reported as showing an 'equivocal' Coombs test and anti-D with some anti-C antibody was identified in the maternal serum. Anti-D gamma globulin was not administered. The husband's Rhesus genotype was assessed as CDe/cde.

In 1987 she was referred to the regional centre for antenatal care in view of the previous history. The anti-D antibody levels at 17, 21 and 28 weeks were 2.35 IU/ml, 2.3 IU/ml, and 2.62 IU/ml respectively with anti-C antibody present but not quantified. Amniocentesis was not performed. The pregnancy continued normally, ultrasound examinations at 28 and 32 weeks confirming normal fetal growth with no signs of hydropic change. At 36 weeks the patient reported the loss of fetal movements. Ultrasound confirmed intrauterine death without any hydramnios, fetal ascites, pleural or pericardial effusions. The maternal antibody level was reported as 370 IU/ml anti-D. Labour was induced and a macerated male fetus of 2500 g was delivered. The placenta weighed 610 g and was macroscopically normal. Autopsy excluded hydropic changes but confirmed extramedullary haemopoiesis consistent with isoimmunization. There were no congenital anomalies.

In the current pregnancy, as the husband was known to be heterozygous for the D antigen, the couple were offered the option of chorion villous biopsy to determine the Rhesus blood group of the fetus. Unable to entertain the option of therapeutic abortion, they elected to carry on with the pregnancy, agreeing to such procedures as necessary should subsequent investigations suggest an affected baby.

At 11 weeks the maternal antibody levels were 282 IU/ml anti-D + anti-C and at 19 weeks 196 IU/ml anti-D + anti-C. Ultrasound at 15 weeks confirmed dates and a normal fetal configuration. At 23 weeks an amniocentesis was performed. The amniotic fluid to bilirubin ratio of 1.275 suggested a severely affected baby. Ultrasound examination at this time confirmed a normally growing fetus with no overt signs of hydrops fetalis.

The patient was referred to a tertiary centre where intrauterine transfusion was accomplished the following day by cordocentesis and repeated subsequently at 24, 26 and 29 weeks. At 48 h after the last procedure the patient was admitted in preterm labour. Labour was suppressed with a ritodrine infusion over a 48-h period. She is now taking oral ritodrine 10 mgm 6-hourly and she has suffered no side-effects from ritodrine apart from occasional palpitations. She is now 30 weeks pregnant.

Questions

Do you consider that there are any anomalies in this history?

There are two. The first pregnancy progressed normally in every way and yet the patient appears to have been sensitized to the C and D antigens by term. The second pregnancy was unusual in that despite levels of antibody that would be consistent either with an unaffected baby or at the worse mild disease it ended with an intrauterine death. Again there were no obstetric complications, e.g. bleeding in pregnancy and the placenta was described as normal without evidence of retroplacental bleeding. There was therefore no explanation for the hundredfold increase in antibody level detected at delivery.

How big a problem is Rhesus isoimmunization?

Although 15% of the Caucasian population are Rhesus negative in the UK very few babies die from the effects of Rhesus isoimmunization, approximately 0.05 per 1000 births.

What factors have been responsible for the improved prognosis in these cases?

The institution of anti-D gammaglobulin prophylaxis for Rhesus negative women bearing Rhesus positive children, the tendency to smaller families, the improved facilities for neonatal intensive care for affected babies and the establishment of referral centres for the investigation and management of such cases.

Describe how you undertake anti-D prophylaxis

All mothers should have their blood group and Rhesus status established at booking. The need is to anticipate when fetal red cells may enter the maternal circulation. This is most likely to happen at delivery. For mothers who are Rhesus negative a sample of cord blood should be taken at delivery, the fetal blood group determined and an indirect Coombs test performed to identify red cell-bound antibody. At the same time a maternal sample is taken for a Kleihauer test to determine the magnitude of any fetomaternal haemorrhage.

Routinely, 500 units i.m. of anti-D gammaglobulin is given as soon as possible after delivery, usually within 24 h, depending upon laboratory practice; however, it can be effective up to 7 days after delivery. The 500 units of anti-D gammaglobulin will neutralize the effect of a 4 ml fetal–maternal blood transfusion equivalent to 160 fetal cells per low power field in a Kleihauer test. If the Kleihauer test suggests a larger fetomaternal transfer then additional anti-D will be required. Such a requirement can occur in association with manual removal of the placenta or at caesarean section.

The prophylactic administration of anti-D is further indicated following either spontaneous or therapeutic abortion in Rhesus negative women. A dose of 250 units is given before 20 weeks and 500 units if more than 20 weeks gestation. Likewise, anti-D should be given following ectopic pregnancy. The same principle applies for antepartum haemorrhage of all kinds. Diagnostic procedures such as chorion villous sampling, amniocentesis, placentocentesis and fetoscopy require prophylaxis as does version for the correction of malpresentation.

Why if prophylaxis is effective do cases continue to present?

Despite established protocols anti-D may have been omitted in a previous pregnancy. The standard dose given might have been insufficient for the degree of fetomaternal bleeding. A transplacental haemorrhage of more than 4 ml occurs in 0.6% of normal deliveries. Sensitization, as in this case, may have occurred undetected early in the first pregnancy. The patient may have had a transfusion as a child which had been forgotten or she may conceal the history of an abortion or a previous pregnancy.

What investigations would you undertake in a case such as this? What treatments might be instituted?

The father is known to be heterozygous for D and therefore there is a 50% chance of this baby being affected. Chorion villous biopsy produces a source of fetal red cells which can be identified as Rhesus D positive by immunofluorescent techniques, thus establishing the Rhesus status of the fetus. The history of a previous stillbirth at 36 weeks resulting from isoimmunization would suggest that in the event of the baby being Rhesus positive then the prognosis would be poor, compromise of the fetus being likely at an even earlier gestation. The identification of a Rhesus positive baby would indicate an early referral to a specialist centre.

In cases where severe disease is a possibility, ultrasound examination of the fetus at weekly intervals is important to identify the early signs of hydropic change.

Estimations of maternal haemolytic antibody should be performed at least every 2 weeks from the outset in a case such as this where the history suggests severe disease. Hydrops and intrauterine death can occur by 20 weeks. Increasing titres of maternal haemolytic antibody usually suggest a deteriorating situation, but a rise in antibody titre can occur when the fetus is Rhesus negative (anamnestic reaction). Titres are less reliable as an index of severity than the quantitative measurement of antibody. When the maternal antibody level remains below 4 IU/ml the degree of fetal haemolysis is likely to be minimal and delivery can be anticipated at term. Antibody levels between 4 IU/ml and 20 IU/ml suggest mild to moderate haemolysis but if the antibody levels rise to 20 IU/ml or more the baby is likely to be severely affected and further investigation is required.

Amniocentesis provides amniotic fluid for the spectrophotometric assay of bilirubin, increasing levels reflecting more fetal haemolysis. The results obtained are plotted on a prediction chart

(Liley) which identifies the severity of the disease and indicates the time when intervention is necessary, be that delivery or intrauterine transfusion. Amniocentesis is only suitable for assessment in the third trimester. When antibody levels are significantly raised in the second trimester fetal blood sampling by cordocentesis enables the severity of fetal anaemia to be ascertained directly.

The history referred to the amniotic fluid to bilirubin ratio. What is this?

The measurement of bilirubin in the amniotic fluid by spectrophotometry is subject to error. The absorption at 450 μm is influenced by the volume of the amniotic fluid, and contamination with blood or meconium. To overcome such effects different indices are adopted by different laboratories. The most commonly used parameter is the linear deviation measuring the peak absorption at 450 μm from a baseline drawn between the readings at 350 μm and 550 μm. The amniotic fluid to bilirubin ratio is an alternative index being the ratio of readings at 520 μm and 490 μm. A bilirubin to protein ratio negates the effects of volume fluctuations both components being diluted or concentrated to the same degree. The greatest care must be taken in interpreting the results from different laboratories especially when patients are transferred from one centre to another.

Cordocentesis is free of these limitations because the assay directly measures the effect of fetal haemolysis by estimating the fetal haemoglobin.

Tell me about intrauterine transfusion?

The purpose of intrauterine transfusion is to correct fetal anaemia, prevent hydropic change and to sustain the baby until delivery. The timing of delivery requires balancing the risks of intrauterine transfusion against those of prematurity. The procedure is initiated by the results of antibody assays, amniocentesis or ultrasound signs of hydropic change. Cordocentesis with a view to intrauterine transfusion may be performed electively 10 weeks before the gestation of a previous stillbirth but not before 18 weeks gestation.

Intrauterine transfusion can be accomplished either by injecting donor blood directly into the fetal peritoneal cavity from which cells are rapidly absorbed into the fetal circulation or directly into a cord vessel by cordocentesis. The donor blood should be fresh, compatible with the mother and packed with the buffy white cell layer removed.

The main determinants of survival for intraperitoneal transfusion are the gestational age at which transfusions are commenced and the state of the fetus at the first transfusion. The outlook for the fetus with hydropic change in early pregnancy is poor possibly because ascites interferes with the absorption of erythrocytes. The timing of subsequent intraperitoneal transfusion is determined by the results of amniocentesis usually at fortnightly intervals.

Cordocentesis is a more direct approach. A transplacental approach is made to an umbilical vessel under ultrasound control. This minimizes the risk of needle displacement by fetal movement. A blood sample is obtained and if the haematocrit or haemoglobin value is below two standard deviations of the mean for gestation, transfusion is commenced directly into the fetal circulation. The volume is determined by consideration of the fetoplacental blood volume, the cord blood haematocrit and the haematocrit of the donor blood. The fetal haematocrit/haemoglobin is measured after transfusion. The timing of subsequent cordocentesis is based on the estimate that the haematocrit will reduce at approximately 1% per day. The procedure is repeated when it is calculated that the haematocrit is in the order of 20–25% or if signs of hydropic change appear on ultrasound.

This patient had a stillbirth in her second pregnancy. What investigations do you undertake when faced with an unexplained stillbirth?

Difficult though it may be for the doctor to ask at a time of anguish for the parents, the patient's permission must be obtained to permit investigation of the fetus to determine the possible cause of death. Even if autopsy is refused it is often possible to obtain permission for more limited biopsy procedures.

The fetus and placenta must be closely examined and the findings recorded. Even negative findings are important, e.g. the absence of retroplacental clot. The fetus should be photographed and copies retained for the parents. If a fresh stillbirth, < 24 h since death, cardiac blood should be aspirated for IgM and IgG levels suggestive of intrauterine infection. The same sample should be used for a fetal TORCH screen (specific antibodies to toxoplasmosis, rubella, cytomegalovirus and herpes simplex). The skin should be swabbed for bacterial culture and if preterm, additional cultures requested for *Chlamydia, Listeria* and *Mycoplasma*. A full-thickness skin and muscle biopsy should be referred for cytogenetic studies. The fetus should be X-rayed before being sent for autopsy. This identifies even mild skeletal anomalies which might indicate some of the rarer inherited disorders.

The placenta should be weighed and bacterial swabs taken from the surface as for the fetus. Amnion should be taken by sterile dissection and sent for cytogenetic analysis. The placenta can then be sent for histological examination.

A maternal blood sample is required for a TORCH screen and repeated 2 weeks later to detect any change in titres in the event of recent infection. A Kleihauer test will identify any significant fetomaternal haemorrhage. Thyroid function tests and the glycosylated haemoglobin concentration will exclude undiagnosed thyroid disease and diabetes. An auto antibody screen will exclude rarer causes of intrauterine loss such as systemic lupus erythematosus.

Discussion

In the red cells almost 250 antigenic factors can be recognized. From the fetal point of view the most important is the Rhesus factor. The Rh blood group is composed of three allelomorphic pairs of genes Cc, Dd and Ee. The main cause of isoimmunization is the D antigen and it is the presence of this antigen which is taken to designate Rhesus positive and towards which prophylaxis with anti-D is directed. The other Rhesus antigens are far less immunogenic but can cause on occasion serious problems. Anti-Kell, anti-Duffy and anti-Kidd antibody can cause haemolytic disease and as the effectiveness of anti-D prophylaxis succeeds so these antigens will assume a higher profile; some laboratories screen for these other blood group antibodies. Sensitization is not an inevitable consequence of pregnancy. Rhesus D negative women giving birth to a Rhesus positive baby have a 7–8% risk of developing antibody within 6 months of delivery and a 17–18% risk of developing antibody in the next pregnancy. In part this is because ABO incompatibility between mother and fetus results in the destruction of the fetal cells before they induce Rh antibody formation. The risk of sensitization following an ABO incompatible pregnancy is only about 12% of that following an ABO compatible pregnancy. In others insufficient fetomaternal transfer occurs to provoke a response although the critical volume appears to vary between individuals.

Although anti-D prophylaxis after delivery has been successful for, as yet, unsensitized Rh(D) negative mothers a small number of women such as this patient develop antibody during the first pregnancy and before delivery. Furthermore, the numbers of new Rh(D) immunizations and of fetal or neonatal deaths have been more or less static over the past decade. In about half the new immunizations the cause is not apparent and therefore it has been suggested that anti-D should be administered to Rhesus negative women during pregnancy to negate this risk. Reductions in the incidence of sensitization have been reported with the administration of 500 IU anti-D immunoglobulin at 28 and 34 weeks gestation. Anti-D immunoglobulin is a valuable commodity and a large multicentre prospective controlled trial is proposed to assess the efficacy of giving of a smaller dose (250 IU) anti-D immunoglobulin at 28 and 34 weeks gestation as prophylaxis in unsensensitized Rhesus negative patients.

Once antibody has been detected, the problem remains to evaluate its effect on the fetus. The presence and level of an antibody titre does not always predict with accuracy the severity of the disease except perhaps in the first affected pregnancy. Consideration of the past history with antibody results allows some prediction as to the likely severity of the disease in a current pregnancy but offers no real guide as to the timing of delivery.

Amniocentesis and amniotic fluid analysis is one step nearer to the fetus but at best is a measure of the products of haemolysis and little is known of the dynamics concerning the transfer of bilirubin into the amniotic fluid. Furthermore, there is a delay between receiving the results and proceeding to intraperitoneal transfusion.

Cordocentesis has the advantage of sampling the fetus directly, and establishing the effects of haemolysis with precision by determining the fetal haemoglobin and haematocrit. The needle can be left *in situ* and intravascular transfusion started immediately if the results of the simple blood test indicate the need. The effects of intravascular transfusion are immediately available at the end of the procedure allowing the timing of the next transfusion to be planned without the imposition of a further assessment by amniocentesis. Earlier intervention may be necessary if ultrasound examination detects hydropic change during the interim. Cordocentesis can be performed with greater reliability than intraperitoneal transfusion in early pregnancy. In the case of the patient presented, cordocentesis at 23 weeks confirmed profound anaemia with a cord haemoglobin of 2.4 g/dl. Thirty ml of donor blood with a haemoglobin of 17 g/dl were transfused and the post-transfusion haemoglobin was 10.0 g/dl.

Another approach might be to remove the offending antibody from the maternal circulation. This would circumvent the complexities of intrauterine manipulation and the complications of such procedures: infection, hepatitis and placental abruption. Plasmapheresis is a technique by which volumes of plasma are removed and replaced with donor plasma. It is only justified in the presence of severe disease. The schedules differ between centres and both small and large volume exchanges have been employed. Resulting hypoproteinaemia can cause gross oedema and with the removal of large amounts of immunoglobulin the patient's resistance to infection can be reduced. Anaemia is also a problem. With increasing concerns about blood products and the success of the newer techniques such therapy is probably contraindicated.

Immune suppression with promethazine and desensitization of the mother by the administration of Rh (D) positive red cell stroma in enteric coated capsules have each been claimed to be of benefit but these results have not been confirmed in subsequent studies.

Comment

The examiner is anxious to establish that the candidate understands the problem presented and that he is constantly aware of when to avoid isoimmunization by the appropriate use of anti-D prophylaxis. As these cases more and more are referred to specialist centres so fewer candidates will have had personal experience of the condition. Therefore, further questioning will reveal the extent of the candidate's reading and interest. It is reasonable that the examiner should ascertain the candidate's comprehension of laboratory results and their significance. Finally, the examiner picks on a small item from the history and switches the discussion to a different topic entirely but one with which the candidate should be entirely familiar.

Outcome

At 31 weeks gestation the patient established in preterm labour. An infusion of ritodrine was again attempted to suppress the uterine activity. At a low rate of infusion the patient complained of severe side-effects with tachycardia and tremors. The infusion was discontinued and she progressed in labour to be delivered 5 h later of a male infant weighing 1.39 kg . The placenta weighed 360 g . The cord blood haemoglobin was 15.5 g/dl. The sample comprised 99% donor blood (A Rhesus negative) and was Coombs negative. Six hours after birth a single exchange transfusion was performed when the bilirubin level was 137 μmol/l. No further management was required.

Further reading

BOWMAN, J. M. (1984) Rhesus haemolytic disease. In *Antenatal and Neonatal Screening* (ed. N. J. Wald) Oxford, Oxford University Press, pp. 314–344

FRASER, I. D., BENNET, M. O., BOTHAMLEY, J. E. and AIRTH, G. R. (1976) Intensive antenatal plasmapheresis in severe rhesus isoimmunisation. *Lancet*, **i**, 6–9

LILEY, A. W. (1961) Liquor amnii analysis in the management of the pregnancy complicated by Rhesus sensitisation. *American Journal of Obstetrics and Gynecology*, **82**, 1359–1370

NICOLAIDES, K. H., SOOTHILL, P. W., RODECK, C. H. and CLEWELL, W. (1986) Rh disease: intravascular fetal blood transfusion by cordocentesis. *Fetal Therapy*, **1**, 185–192

Case 20

A 22-year-old married canteen worker was referred to the gynaecological clinic because of secondary infertility. Two years before she had been delivered normally of a male infant after an uneventful pregnancy. The third stage was uncomplicated. This had been a planned pregnancy and the patient had fallen pregnant soon after discontinuing barrier contraception with condoms. There were no problems during the puerperium. Breast feeding was established and continued for 8 months. A low oestrogen combined oral contraceptive was taken from 6 weeks postpartum. This preparation was discontinued 3 months after her baby was weaned from the breast. The patient noticed persistent discharge from the left breast and a more intermittent loss from the right. The discharge was milky in colour and had never been bloodstained. After stopping the oral contraceptive her cycle failed to establish. She was also anxious that although wanting another child her 'sex drive' was almost non-existent. Intercourse was painful and sore. There was nothing of significance in her medical or family history and she was taking no medication. She complained of no visual disturbance. She denied manual expression of the milk.

On examination she was of normal stature and appropriate weight. She was normotensive, BP 110/70 mmHg. There was no goitre. The breasts were normal to palpation. There was no supraclavicular or axillary lymphadenopathy. It was possible to express milk from both nipples. The hair distribution was normal and female. On pelvic examination the external genitalia looked normal but speculum examination was uncomfortable and the vaginal skin appeared thin and atrophic. There was no cervical mucus and the uterus felt rather small for a parous patient.

Questions

What is your initial diagnosis?

Secondary infertility with secondary amenorrhoea and galactorrhoea.

Yes, but what pathology might be responsible for this picture?

Hyperprolactinaemia.

What causes of hyperprolactinaemia are you aware of?

The secretion of prolactin is regulated by a short negative feedback control system involving an hypothalamic prolactin release inhibiting hormone (PRIH). Drugs which interfere with the synthesis, storage or action of PRIH may be responsible. Such drugs include dopamine, reserpine or dopamine antagonists like the phenothiazines or metoclopramide. Cimetidine may also have an effect but usually only in high dosage. Hyperprolactinaemia may also present in association with primary hypothyroidism. The prolactin secreting cells of the pituitary gland are situated in the lateral portions of the gland. Hypersecretion may be associated with hyperplasia or adenoma formation. Prolactinomas smaller than 1 cm in diameter are designated as microadenomas.

How would you deal with a case of drug-induced hyperprolactinaemia?

It would depend on the indication for the drug in the first place. For the resolution of her symptoms the patient would be best served by discontinuing the treatment or changing to an alternative.

However, it might not be appropriate to discontinue psychotropic drugs for example, in which case it might be necessary to add a dopamine agonist such as bromocriptine to her medication. There is in fact no clear answer to the question, so much depends on the balance between the symptomatology from the effects of hyperprolactinaemia and the underlying problem.

How would you proceed in the evaluation of this case?

The patient is not menstruating and therefore attention must be directed first to the assessment of the pituitary-ovarian axis bearing in mind the probability of hyperprolactinaemia and its various causes. Evaluation of the husband is unlikely to be productive but a sperm count should be requested. If for any reason the seminal analysis is deficient then that result might modify the pursuit of the fertility problem, especially if surgery or prolonged medical treatment is envisaged. I would request serum gonadotrophin, prolactin and oestradiol levels. In addition I would ask for thyroid function tests and a lateral X-ray of the skull.

How would you interpret these results?

FSH:	3.0 U/l	LH:	2.0 U/l
17-beta-oestradiol:	60 pmol/l	Progesterone:	< 5 nmol/l
Prolactin:	2320 mU/l	T4:	80 nmol/l
T3:	2.1 nmol/l	TSH:	4.3 mU/l
Thyroglobulin:	68 μg/l	RBS:	4.3 mmol/l
Lateral skull X-ray:	Normal		

The gonadotrophin levels are within normal limits but presumably are not being secreted in the normal sequential pattern. Prolactin also has a peripheral effect antagonizing the effects of FSH and LH at the ovarian level. The beta-oestradiol level, however, is depressed which fits in with the hypo-oestrogenic picture on clinical examination and her symptoms of dyspareunia. The report for progesterone is ambiguous and presumably represents levels below the sensitivity of the assay. The prolactin level is raised and a third of such patients harbour a prolactinoma. She is euthyroid and a random blood sugar level is normal. The normal lateral skull X-ray does not exclude an adenoma of the pituitary gland.

What is the next step?

The hypo-oestrogenic status could be confirmed by either a negative progesterone challenge test or curettage which would yield only scanty inactive endometrium. The serum prolactin level is not grossly raised and elevated levels can be recorded at times of stress. The result should be confirmed by inserting a fine butterfly needle into a peripheral vein and taking half hour samples with the patient at rest. If elevated levels fall to normal over the test period then a response to stress is the most likely explanation of the initial result. If the level is sustained then hyperprolactinaemia is confirmed.

If hyperprolactinaemia is confirmed then it is important to exclude the presence of a prolactinoma within the pituitary gland. The pituitary fossa should be imaged with high definition CT scanning. Adenomas are characterized by hypodense areas, often asymmetrical, within the gland and with deviation of the pituitary stalk. There may be variable degrees of bony erosion in the sella floor or enlargement of the pituitary fossa. Further management depends on the situation of an adenoma, its size and position. If a prolactinoma extends above the diaphragma sella then it can compress the optic chiasma to produce a degree of bitemporal hemianopia. The patient can be quite unaware of this complication in the early stages and an assessment of the visual fields is mandatory when pituitary adenomata are suspected.

This patient's CT scan confirmed a microadenoma in the right side of the pituitary gland. There is no visual field defect. Have you any ideas as to her future management?

To some degree that will depend on whether, in the knowledge that the problem exists and what the options are, the patient elects to pursue a pregnancy or simply to seek relief of her symptoms of oestrogen deficiency and galactorrhoea.

If the patient chooses not to go in for a pregnancy then her symptoms can be relieved by prescribing bromocriptine to reduce the prolactin levels to normal. Ovulatory cycles should ensue, adequate oestrogenization of the genital tract follow and her libido return. Her galactorrhoea will also disappear. Low doses (2.5–5.0 mg/day) are usually sufficient to maintain the prolactin level within normal values; higher doses may be required to produce ovulatory cycles. Should she fall pregnant on this regimen then the drug should be discontinued as soon as possible after conception. It would need to be reintroduced following confinement as her symptoms will recur. Alternatively transsphenoidal microadenomectomy might at the outset cure her. The choice of treatment for this symptomatic relief can only be established after discussion between the patient, the gynaecologist and the neurosurgeon.

What if she still wishes to become pregnant?

Pregnancy is associated with an enlargement of the pituitary gland. The prolactinoma itself may also grow. The concern is that such enlargement upwards might precipitate headache with impaired visual acuity and restriction of the visual fields, or if growth is lateral the development of a cavernous sinus syndrome. These sequelae can become permanent. Surgical extirpation of a prolactinoma has been thought to be advisable before embarking on a pregnancy. Microadenomas and laterally placed macroadenomas can usually be dealt with by a transphenoidal approach. This operation leaves no scar and requires only a short hospital stay. Macroadenomas with extension upwards demand the more extensive transfrontal adenectomy. The removal of these larger tumours may cause hypopituitarism. In such cases gonadotrophin therapy will be necessary to achieve a pregnancy.

Discussion

Hyperprolactinaemia is not uncommon. Raised prolactin levels are found in one in five cases of women presenting with amenorrhoea. In 40% of these there is a detectable pituitary tumour. Microadenomas are more common than macroadenomas.

It is now well established that bromocriptine therapy can achieve a dramatic shrinkage in size for even large macroadenomata. The role of surgery before embarking on a pregnancy remains an item for debate. The fear is that further enlargement of an adenoma and the pituitary in pregnancy might result in permanent neurological sequelae including blindness. On the other hand, if the dimensions of the tumour can be significantly reduced by medical means first, then in an ensuing pregnancy there might be sufficient space to accommodate the inevitable enlargement of the pituitary fossa contents without causing neurological sequelae. Surgery would then be reserved for those patients where tumour regression had been considered insufficient on medical treatment. The hesitation about surgery stems from the risk of subsequent hypopituitarism which would further impair the patient's fertility, and also the unpredictable outcome of surgery. The surgical treatment of microadenomas produces ovulatory cycles in 80% of patients but for macroadenomas the success rate is only 40%. The failures in both groups would still require bromocriptine after surgery to normalize prolactin levels and induce ovulation.

The central role for bromocriptine therapy implies, for some patients, long-term therapy. The evidence is that once remission has been achieved, maintenance therapy is possible on very low doses and that the therapy is well tolerated. Finally, when treatment is eventually discontinued although prolactin levels may rise, the adenomas do not recur.

There has accumulated in the literature evidence that neurological sequelae are rare when pregnancy follows bromocriptine therapy for surgically untreated prolactinomas. The risk may be as little as 2% for microadenomas and therefore to advise surgery as a necessary prelude to pregnancy is excessive. Bromocriptine can be given as primary therapy to achieve pregnancy in such cases. The drug is discontinued at conception. There is no evidence of a teratogenic risk to the fetus but it can cross the placenta and reduce prolactin levels in the fetus. The patient is urged to report any headache or visual disturbance to the clinic immediately. The visual fields should be assessed at each visit to the hospital. However, tumour expansion can be very rapid. Should the signs of neurological involvement develop, then if the baby is sufficiently mature, delivery should be accomplished. Failing that, large doses of bromocriptine might achieve some regression of the tumour. Dexamethasone can reduce intracranial pressure as well as fetal pulmonary maturity for early delivery. In the final event surgical decompression may be necessary.

The case for primary bromocriptine therapy for macroadenomas with a view to pregnancy has been less precise. Early reports suggested that neurological sequelae and tumour growth were common when pregnancy occurred in the presence of a macroadenoma and even that these complications were more likely to develop if the macroadenoma had been treated with bromocriptine first. This work has been reappraised and the point made that in the cases quoted there was no evidence that any tumour shrinkage had occurred before pregnancy had supervened. The identification of tumour regression is essential before pregnancy is to be encouraged. When this provision is fulfilled the prognosis for the patient in a pregnancy is excellent.

The picture has emerged that bromocriptine is the treatment of choice for prolactinomas of all sizes in the first instance. Once tumour regression has been identified pregnancy can be permitted. Surgery is reserved for those patients where medical treatment fails. Surgery should be selective to avoid hypopituitarism.

The causes of pituitary prolactinomas are unknown. Because treatment with oestrogen is known to stimulate prolactin secretion the increased use of the oral contraceptive has been suggested as the reason for an increase in the numbers of cases diagnosed in recent years. This apparent effect has much more to do with the increased awareness of gynaecologists that any menstrual disturbance can be caused by hyperprolactinaemia and therefore there has been more recourse to serum prolactin estimations in the evaluation of these cases. When cases of amenorrhoea and galactorrhoea or amenorrhoea and hyperprolactinaemia are analysed with respect to oral contraceptive usage there is no excess of prolactinomas in women who previously used the oral contraceptive.

Outcome

This patient elected to undergo transphenoidal microadenomectomy as a primary procedure. The operation was straightforward and she was hospitalized for only 4 days. Four months later her menstrual cycle was well established and prolactin levels were normal. She then fell pregnant. The pregnancy and delivery were normal. Breast feeding was established and maintained for 6 months after which there was no galactorrhoea, her prolactin levels remained normal and normal menstruation again supervened.

Comment

With symptoms involving the breast, the candidate should make a point when reporting his findings on examination, to emphasize that the possibility of breast carcinoma has been considered.

The candidate was correct at the outset to be cautious, keeping his options open when asked for a diagnosis. Too rapid a commitment can lead to disastrous results if his diagnosis is wrong. The examiner made it clear quickly enough that a decision was what he wanted and the candidate responded.

When discussing management, especially when there are options and there is no overall agreement within the profession, it is appropriate to mention counselling the patient and seeking her opinion. This should be merely a reflection of good practice in any event. Informed consent by the patient is a statutory requirement.

Further reading

TAN, S. L. and JACOBS, H. S. (1986) Management of prolactinomas – 1986. *British Journal of Obstetrics and Gynaecology*, **93**, 1025–1029

Case 21

The patient is 27 years of age, single and unemployed. She is in her second pregnancy. The first in 1986 was entirely normal. She was delivered at 39 weeks gestation of a healthy boy weighing 3113 g. Her past medical history is unremarkable. She neither smokes nor drinks. Her mother is diabetic but this has been attributed to long-term steroid therapy for asthma.

She booked in hospital for the current pregnancy with a history of 12 weeks amenorrhoea. The LMP had been carefully recorded and she had a regular menstrual cycle, 5/28. She had been using sheaths for contraception, on her own admission, somewhat intermittently. On clinical examination the uterine size was consistent with dates and her general examination was satisfactory. Blood tests confirmed that she was not anaemic (Hb 13.3 g/dl), that her blood group was A Rhesus positive, she was immune to rubella and that screening for specific disease was negative. A random blood sugar level was 5.1 mmol/l.

Ultrasound examination at 17 weeks confirmed a singleton pregnancy. The BPD was 3.6 cm and the femur length 20 mm. There appeared to be no fetal abnormalities. The placenta was described as being posterior in position but extending down and thinly covering the os. The findings were recorded in her shared care documentation and arrangements were made for her to continue her antenatal care with her GP, and to be seen again in the hospital clinic at 33 weeks gestation for a repeat ultrasound examination.

The patient was referred to the hospital as an emergency by her GP at 31 weeks gestation. Shortly after her last visit to the hospital she had some slight bleeding per vaginum. She was advised to rest by her GP and the bleeding subsided. Her antenatal care had then continued satisfactorily. When seen by him at 31 weeks she reported that all had been well and in answer to direct questioning denied any vaginal bleeding.

On the night of admission she had called her GP because of fresh bright bleeding per vaginum in bed. The loss had amounted to a couple of tablespoonfuls and had been unprovoked. It was sufficient however to substantially stain her nightdress and the bedding. She denied pain and discomfort at the time but confessed to backache and lower abdominal discomfort during the day. There appeared to be no active bleeding and her transfer was arranged to hospital by her GP via a standard ambulance.

In hospital her history changed somewhat. She admitted to episodes of bright red 'show' on several occasions from 26 weeks. She had denied the possibility for fear of referral to hospital because of difficulties in making arrangements for her child. There had also been some bleeding in association with the abdominal discomfort she had experienced the day before admission. She felt also that fetal movements might have been reduced over this period. It also transpired that her partner, who had left the home earlier in the pregnancy, had returned and that coitus had taken place on the night of admission although she denied any such activity in association with the earlier losses.

She was not shocked and did not require blood transfusion. There has been no more bleeding since admission. Blood tests have been undertaken and an ultrasound examination repeated. She has been advised to stay in hospital until the delivery of her baby.

She is now 34 weeks pregnant by dates. She is not clinically anaemic. The uterine size is consistent with the period of amenorrhoea. The uterus is soft and not irritable on palpation. A single fetus occupies a longitudinal lie but the presenting, part i.e. the head is clearly palpated high above the pelvic brim and freely mobile. The baby does not feel unduly small and there does not appear to be excess amniotic fluid present. There was no uterine tenderness present. The patient's sanitary towel is unstained.

Questions

What is your diagnosis?

Threatened abortion and recurrent antepartum haemorrhage.

What is the probable cause?

The history is confused and has not been consistent. The silent presentation at this gestation, the recurrent and self-limiting nature of the bleeding and the palpation of the fetal head high out of the pelvis would suggest a placenta praevia. However, the episode of backache and lower abdominal discomfort preceding the bleed that occasioned her admission is associated with a posterior placenta and could suggest a degree of abruption at that site.

What causes of antepartum haemorrhage do you recognize?

Antepartum haemorrhage is defined as bleeding from the genital tract after 28 weeks gestation. The definition therefore includes bleeding from local lesions in the lower genital tract such as vaginitis, cervical polyps, cervicitis, cervical and vaginal varices, and malignant lesions of the vagina or cervix. Such local causes account for only 5% of cases. Haemorrhage from placental or fetal vessels is more significant and includes bleeding from placenta praevia, abruptio placentae, vasa praevia, marginal separation and circumvallate placentae. The last three are usually diagnosed retrospectively. For practical purposes clinical examination and ultrasound evaluation identify bleeding from placenta praevia, abruptio placentae and by exclusion bleeding of unknown aetiology.

How would you rank these in terms of their threat to the fetus?

Abruptio placentae, bleeding of unknown origin and placenta praevia.

How important is antepartum haemorrhage from the point of view of maternal mortality?

Antepartum haemorrhage is a rare cause of maternal death. The report on confidential enquiries into maternal deaths in England and Wales for the triennium 1982–1984 listed only 4 cases: 2 placenta praevia and 2 abruptio placentae, representing a 60% reduction over a decade. The report did emphasize the predictable risk of severe haemorrhage at caesarean section in women with a history of previous caesarean section in whom the placenta is anterior and low lying. In such cases the placenta may be morbidly adherent to the lower segment scar and caesarean section may have to be followed by hysterectomy. Caesarean section for placenta praevia should only be undertaken by senior staff or under their direct supervision. The report also reiterated the need for each unit to have an established protocol to deal with massive haemorrhage.

What would be your management from this point on?

The early ultrasound examination suggested a low lying placenta. Routine scanning in the early second trimester identifies a low lying placenta in 6% of cases. Of these, 6% will have a persisting placenta praevia at 30–32 weeks. A repeat ultrasound examination is required to confirm the clinical diagnosis and possibly to identify evidence of any retroplacental bleeding. If the latter were identified then a less conservative approach would be adopted in the event of any further loss.

The patient should stay in hospital even if placenta praevia is excluded. The history is of at least two episodes of vaginal bleeding and even if this is bleeding of unknown aetiology multiple episodes suggest a significant risk for the fetus.

The wellbeing of the fetus should be assessed by the implementation of a daily fetal movement record, daily recording of the fetal cardiotogram, and serial ultrasound examinations to identify any development of IUGR.

The mother is Rhesus positive and therefore anti-D administration is not required. However, there may have been a significant fetomaternal haemorrhage that could evoke other antibody formation. Cross-matched blood needs to be available at all times but the cross-match needs to be repeated weekly in case the mother's immune status has changed.

Bedrest is advised initially until all bleeding has stopped for 2 days after which mobilization should be encouraged to reduce the risk of deep vein thrombosis. A gentle speculum examination could then be performed to exclude a local cause for the bleeding if placenta praevia has been excluded.

The mother must not be allowed to become anaemic and her haemoglobin should be maintained at normal levels by haematinics and if necessary by transfusion.

If placenta praevia is confirmed and the home unit lacks facilities for the care of the preterm baby then intrauterine transfer to a unit with such facilities should be considered once the maternal situation has been stabilized. Further bleeding might precipitate the need for urgent delivery and transit is contraindicated in the presence of haemorrhage.

How and when would you deliver this patient?

If placenta praevia were positively excluded on ultrasound I would allow the patient to go into spontaneous labour. The perinatal mortality in such cases is increased because of preterm labour and delivery rather than placental insufficiency. Should the tests of fetal well-being imply fetal compromise then induction of labour would be indicated if the fetus were sufficiently mature, otherwise delivery by caesarean section would be more appropriate.

If the problem is placenta praevia of a major degree as defined by ultrasound then delivery is by caesarean section. The timing will depend upon a number of factors. Delivery would be precipitated by a deterioration in fetal well-being. In the event of further bleeding either further conservative management or delivery would be implemented depending on the magnitude of the loss and the availability of neonatal services.

The operation should be undertaken when the appropriate expertise is present. A lower segment incision is advisable except when the lower segment has failed to form or the placenta is anterior and the lower segment excessively vascular, in which case a vertical incision starting in the lower segment can be employed. Particular care must be taken not to tear the lower segment during the extraction of the fetus. If the placenta is encountered beneath the incision then it should be separated off the uterine wall until the membranes are encountered and ruptured. Incision of or tearing through the placenta may result in profound fetal blood loss. Likewise the cord should be clamped immediately following delivery to reduce fetal haemorrhage through the placenta.

If there is any doubt as to the site of the placenta or if facilities do not exist for ultrasound placental localization then there remains the option of excluding placenta praevia by digital exploration with the patient anaesthetized in theatre at 37–38 weeks. The attendant staff must be scrubbed and ready to proceed should haemorrhage be precipitated by the examination. Epidural anaesthesia is contraindicated under such circumstances because of the problem of volume replacement in a vasodilated patient and the inevitable anxiety to the mother when she is aware of an emergency situation.

What do you think were the blood tests taken at the time of her admission?

Haemoglobin estimation, cross-matching, Kleihauer test, clotting screen including fibrin degradation products.

The clotting screen was normal but the test for fibrin degradation products was mildly positive (0.7 mg/l) and the Kleihauer test reported one fetal red cell per 200 000 maternal cells. The ultrasound examination confirmed a posterior placenta, the lower edge just reaching the internal cervical os.

Those results would suggest that there was an element of placental separation in association with a grade 2 placenta praevia.

Discussion

Vellamentous insertion of the cord is commonly associated with a low lying placenta. There is a risk of damage to the unprotected fetal vessels which produces sometimes fatal haemorrhage. Bleeding from placenta praevia is principally from the uterine wall at the site of shearing but in some cases there will be a fetal component. In those babies which die *in utero* following bleeding from placenta praevia the findings of fetal anaemia, compensatory erythropoiesis and villous hyperplasia suggest that fetal haemorrhage has occurred. The diagnosis is usually made after birth by inspection of the fetal membranes or the delivery of an anaemic infant. A small APH associated with fetal distress in the absence of signs suggestive of abruption should alert the obstetrician to the possibility of fetal bleeding. Blood from the vaginal haemorrhage should be collected and 2–3 drops added to a test tube half filled with a 1% aqueous solution of sodium hydroxide. The tube is shaken and allowed to stand for 90 s. A brown-green solution indicates haemolysis of maternal red cells, a red-pink solution the presence of fetal cells which have resisted denaturation with alkali. A control tube with maternal venous blood should be used for comparison.

Massive haemorrhage is always a risk with placenta praevia either antenatally or at delivery. It is essential that in every unit there should be an agreed procedure for the management of such haemorrhage with which the medical, midwifery, nursing, laboratory and portering staff are fully conversant.

There is no test which can be applied to establish the well-being of the fetus *in utero* and therefore several are employed in the hope that one will reveal fetal compromise should the others fail to do so. The tendency is to intervene 'to play safe' when one test is adverse, ignoring the reassuring results of other tests. Such intervention can be contrary to the welfare of the fetus.

No method of assessment will predict sudden events such as abruption or cord prolapse following rupture of the membranes. From the fetal standpoint the purpose of antenatal assessment is primarily to avoid antepartum stillbirth and fetal hypoxia and to detect IUGR. When a risk is identified prompt intervention is designed to pre-empt intrapartum death, fetal distress in labour, birth asphyxia, neonatal death and morbidity and long-term problems such as cerebral palsy and mental impairment.

There is a clear association between reduced fetal movement counts and antepartum death but controlled trials indicate that the technique of fetal movement recording has a higher negative predictive value than positive, i.e. the test is less successful in identifying the fetus at risk than the fetus that is well.

On the basis that the placenta is an integral part of the fetoplacental unit many biochemical tests have been instituted to assess 'placental function' in the hope that compromise in the fetus would be reflected in changes in the biochemical parameters. Oestrogens (total, oestriol, oestriol conjugates, etc.), human placental lactogen (HPL), alpha-fetoprotein (AFP), human chorionic gonadotrophin (HCG), progestogens, placental proteins (Schwangerschaftsprotein-1, pregnancy-associated plasma protein A), and placental enzymes (alkaline phosphatase, diamine oxidase, oxytocinase) have all had their enthusiastic proponents.

When the published material is critically assessed, apart from early pregnancy and screening for fetal abnormalities, biochemical tests are of little value for the general care of individual women. For the majority of indications in the second half of pregnancy when a test of fetal well-being is required, biochemical tests represent a waste of scarce resources.

Attention has therefore been directed to fetal assessment by physical measurements: cardiotocography, real-time ultrasound and Doppler measurements of fetal blood flow.

Continuous fetal heart rate monitoring in labour has been used to identify the fetus at risk for asphyxia. The same technique can be applied antenatally with or without uterine stimulation (stress testing). Stress testing is best avoided. Severe fetal heart rate abnormalities may be precipitated and uterine tetany is a possibility. The technique is not appropriate in association with antepartum haemorrhage, preterm labour, premature rupture of the membranes or placenta praevia, all categories where evaluation of the fetus is desirable.

The non-stress test, essentially the evaluation of a fetal heart trace without uterine stimulation, has been widely adopted but no standards have been established for the conduct of the test. The duration of the test, the frequency of testing and the gestational ages at which the results are considered valid differ from report to report. Because of artefact up to 15% of records are unsatisfactory for interpretation. It is generally agreed that the trace should be inspected to determine the basal fetal heart rate, the baseline variability, and the presence or absence of decelerations or accelerations associated with fetal movements or spontaneous uterine activity. However, whether the traces are 'eyeballed' or scored, there remains significant intra- and interobserver variation. Scoring does improve the correlation with adverse outcome.

Fetal biophysical profiles carry the principle of scoring to other fetal attributes determined by ultrasound. Fetal breathing movements, fetal movements, fetal tone and fetal reactivity are assessed and an estimate made of the maximum dimension of the amniotic fluid pool. Some of the criteria are very subjective and yet little is known of the reproducibility of the test. The detailed ultrasound examination required does allow for the identification of unexpected fetal anomalies which might modify the management of the case. It would seem that biophysical profiles do offer a higher specificity for abnormal results than the non-stress test.

Doppler wave form analysis to identify anomalies of fetal blood flow, e.g. the absence of end diastolic flow in the fetal aorta or cord vessels remains largely a research tool. Abnormal results appear to correlate well with adverse outcome.

In many ways the current position resembles the situation when so many placental function tests were the fashion. It is one thing to demonstrate the predictive value of an investigation in terms of its association with some measure of fetal outcome, and quite another to translate that into practice. Because no single test has been shown to discriminate absolutely in defining the fetus in peril from the healthy fetus more and more tests are being combined to produce hopefully better indices of fetal well-being. In the end the only analysis that matters is a truly randomized trial utilizing the test to determine management and to assess the benefit if any. To date this information is not available and tests of clinical well-being should only be used as an adjunct to clinical judgement.

Comment

The history that a patient gives a candidate may differ from that in the possession of the examiner. The examiners are aware of this and will sometimes clarify with the patient the situation should the difference in the records be significant. The patient knowing that she is in an examination situation may be tempted to withhold information. In giving the history the candidate can state what specific questions were asked and what the patient's response was if he considers the information withheld important to the interpretation of the case.

Despite the quality of the history given, the story of vaginal bleeding at this gestation and the findings on clinical examination lead to an almost unavoidable diagnosis. The result of the definitive investigation, the ultrasound examination, was purposely withheld by the examiner. The examiner may do this to assess the candidate's ability to keep all possible options under consideration when planning the management of the patient.

Obligatory reading for this examination must be the *Confidential Enquiries into Maternal Deaths in England and Wales.* Questions on its content can emerge in any phase of the examination. The recommendations within the Report have done much to fashion modern practice and to establish the standards of pregnancy care. Candidates will be expected to be fully conversant with its content.

There is no equivalent national document for perinatal mortality but several regions have established their own surveys. The candidate should be familiar with these and if they are not available be able to quote figures from his own unit.

Outcome

The patient remained in hospital until 38 weeks when an elective lower segment caesarean section was performed to deliver a healthy male infant of 3010 g. There were no further episodes of bleeding. At operation a grade 2 placenta praevia was confirmed. There was no overt evidence of antepartum placental separation.

Further reading

ALEXANDER, S., STANWELL-SMITH, R., BUEKENS, P. and KEIRSE, M. J. N. C. (1989) Biochemical assessment of fetal well-being. In *Effective Care in Pregnancy and Childbirth* (ed. I. Chalmers., M. Enkin and M. J. N. C. Kierse). Oxford, Oxford University Press, pp. 455–471

Department of Health (1989) Report on Health and Social Subjects, 34, *Report on Confidential Enquiries into Maternal Deaths in England and Wales* 1982–1984. HMSO, London, pp. 20–28, 29–30, 137, 149

MANNING, F. A., MORRISON, I., LANGE, I. R., HARMAN, C. R. and CHAMBERLAIN, P. F. (1985) Fetal assessment based on fetal biophysical profile scoring:experience in 12 620 referred high risk pregnancies. American Journal of Obstetrics and Gynecology, **151**, 343–350

RUPARELIA, B. A. and CHAPMAN, M. G. (1985) Early low lying placentae – ultrasonic assessment, progress and outcome. *European Journal of Obstetrics, Gynaecology and Reproductive Biology*, **20**, 209–213

WILLOCKS, J. (1971) Antepartum haemorrhage of uncertain origin. *Journal of Obstetrics and Gynaecology*, **78**, 987–991

Case 22

The 71-year-old retired cleaner was refered to the casualty department by her GP as an emergency with profuse vaginal bleeding. She had reported some loss a month before but this had resolved somewhat after he had prescribed tranexamic acid for her. On the day of admission she had flooded, passing large clots. There was no pain. Her menopause had been at 51 years of age. She had not had intercourse for several years. She had no recollection of ever having a cervical smear. She was known to have angina for 2–3 years and she rapidly became breathless on exertion. She was orthopnoeic requiring two or three pillows to sleep at night. She was aware that she had lost 3 stones in weight over the past 18 months. As a young woman she had pulmonary tuberculosis but this had been treated and she was no longer under any review. Twenty years ago she had had a cholecystectomy and exploration of the common bile duct. She had two children aged 45 and 38 years. The pregnancies and deliveries had been uncomplicated. Her medication included atenolol 100 mg once daily, chlorthalidone 25 mg once daily, and an iron and multivitamin preparation.

On examination she was 155 cm tall and obese weighing 78.2 kg. She looked pale and ill and was slow to answer questions. Her hair was dry and she was somewhat coarse featured. Her BP was 160/80 mmHg. The pulse was 60 beats/min slow and regular, her right radial pulse was smaller in volume than the left. There was a faint systolic ejection murmur maximal over the aortic area, a right carotid bruit and a right subclavian bruit. The apex was displaced suggesting cardiac enlargement. There were no signs of cardiac failure. There was poor chest expansion but air entry was equal on both sides, the breath sounds were vesicular and there were a few scattered rhonchi but no crepitations. The breasts were normal.

The abdomen was obese but soft. The liver was not palpable. There were scars from a previous Kocher's incision and a right upper paramedian incision.

The vulva was atrophic. A speculum examination confirmed a lax vagina and a normal-looking cervix. There was no active bleeding but old blood was present in the cervical canal and in the vagina. The cervix was gently wiped free of blood and a cervical smear taken. Bimanual examination was unhelpful. Because of the obesity it was impossible to define the uterine size or any adnexal pathology.

Her haemoglobin was 10.8 g/dl with an MCV of 85 fl, the white cell count was 10.8×10^9/l. The plasma urea and electrolytes, including potassium, were within normal limits. Thyroid function tests confirmed myxoedema. The ECG showed some ischaemic changes consistent with an old anterior infarction and with sinus bradycardia. A random blood glucose level was 7.9 mmol/l. Urinalysis was normal. A pelvic ultrasound examination confirmed a uniformly enlarged uterus. The cavity was expanded and contained echoes consistent with blood clot and debris. There was no ovarian enlargement. Her cervical smear was reported as atrophic but negative.

The patient was taken to theatre 48 h later for examination under an anaesthetic and curettage. The uterus was certainly enlarged but even under anaesthetic it was impossible to define its limits manually. It appeared to be mobile. There was no adnexal swelling. The cervix was patulous and clot could be seen protruding through the os. Curettage of the endocervical canal yielded only a few fragments. The uterine cavity was cautiously sounded to 8 cm. Curettage confirmed a wide expanded cavity. Necrotic tumour was obtained from all surfaces but nowhere did it encroach on the isthmus. Curettage provoked heavy bleeding and the patient received three units of blood in theatre. Cystoscopy and sigmoidoscopy to 18 cm were normal. The endocervical curettings were reported to be free of any tumour. The endometrial curettings confirmed poorly differentiated adenocarcinoma showing evidence of invasion into the underlying myometrium. There was extensive necrosis.

Following the diagnostic D and C a glucose tolerance test was performed and it confirmed impaired glucose tolerance. A chest X-ray and IVU were normal as was a CT scan for secondary deposits.

Four days after the diagnostic procedure the patient was again taken to theatre for the insertion of intracavity and vaginal caesium.

She tolerated the procedure well. She remained in hospital for a further 3 weeks during which her vaginal loss virtually disappeared. She was then discharged home on a diet and with treatment for her hypothyroidism. Now, 3 weeks later, she has been readmitted for further surgery. During the interim she has felt much better.

Questions

This lady as you have been told has endometrial carcinoma. She has received preoperative treatment with caesium. Have you any observations to make about the initial management?

Total hysterectomy with bilateral oophorectomy or radical hysterectomy are the keystones of management for carcinoma of the endometrium when growth is limited to the corpus or to the corpus and cervix. The place of adjuvant radiotherapy either before or after surgery is less clear when long-term survival is considered. In this case however the gynaecologist was faced with a dilemma. The patient had presented with a considerable haemorrhage. It was imperative to establish the diagnosis and this resulted in further heavy bleeding. She was not a fit woman. She had a known cardiac history and was symptomatic from this point of view. It was discovered that her glucose tolerance was impaired and that she was hypothyroid. Surgery was still ultimately desirable but delay might have resulted in catastrophic haemorrhage during the interim. The insertion of caesium therefore would not only be an adjunct to the surgery but also a first aid measure to reduce the tumour bulk and lessen the risk of haemorrhage while the patient was being further investigated and made fit for surgery.

We are told that she received a total radiation dose of 50 Gy to point A. What is the significance of this statement?

Following the insertion of the intracavity container and vaginal ovoids but before loading the isotope, X-rays are taken of the pelvis which enable the physicist to plot contours representing radiation dosage at progressive distances from the sources. Point A is estimated to be 2 cm above the vaginal vault and 2 cm lateral to the cervix. It represents the site of the ureter which is vulnerable to radiation damage. The dose of isotope inserted and the duration of treatment is designed to deliver a cancericidal dose of radiation to the tumour while safeguarding the ureter. One Gy is equivalent to 100 rads and therefore this patient received 5000 rads at point A. For carcinoma of the cervix higher doses would be delivered but this represents a cancericidal dose for the endometrium.

What contraindications might there be in a case such as this to primary radiation therapy?

Any active inflammatory process within the pelvis such as diverticulitis, active pelvic sepsis or pyometra. Significant old pelvic infection such as a pelvic abscess where bowel might be secured by adhesions. Any coexistent abdominal or adnexal mass including a pelvic kidney. The presence of ascites.

What are the usual sites of recurrence after surgery?

The commonest site is at the vaginal vault. This probably represents lymphatic spread. The pelvic lymph nodes are a common site of recurrence. Occasionally secondaries develop in the lower vagina probably representing haematological spread. Likewise distant metastases to liver, lung, bowel and bone occur more frequently by this route than for cervical carcinoma where spread is overwhelmingly by lymphatics.

Do you know of any variations in technique that might reduce the dissemination of the tumour at surgery?

On the grounds that implantation of malignant cells at the vault may occur after spillage through the cervix during surgery it is advised that the cervical canal be plugged with ribbon gauze soaked in alcohol at the start of the procedure. The chances are, however, that the cells are already in the vault lymphatics at the time of surgery. Postoperative vault radiation has been shown to reduce the incidence of vault recurrence. Others advocate that the removal of a cuff of vagina is mandatory but the efficacy of this in preventing vault recurrence is not established. It has been suggested that the tubes should be ligatured close to the uterus before hysterectomy to prevent spillage of cells into the peritoneum by that route as a result of handling the uterus during the operation. Apart from the use of postoperative vault irradiation there is no objective evidence that these manoeuvres are of any real benefit.

What factors influence the outcome of treatment in endometrial carcinoma?

Primarily the staging of the disease. Until recently this was based on the preoperative clinical assessment, but more recently FIGO have advised a staging based on the surgical findings which, it is maintained, relates more precisely to the ultimate prognosis. Under the earlier classification Stage I disease (carcinoma limited to the corpus) had a 74% 5 year survival rate. When the growth involved the cervix (Stage II) as it does in approximately 10% of cases the 5-year survival rate dropped to 57%. Extension within the confines of the pelvis (Stage III) was associated with a 29% 5-year survival rate but further extension or involvement of the bladder or rectum resulted in only a 9% survival rate to 5 years. A major concern was defining, before definitive surgery, whether the disease involved the cervix. Fractional curettage is a crude tool for this purpose and consequently the incidence of Stage II disease differs widely between centres.

Progressive lack of differentiation in the endometrium is related to the depth of penetration into the myometrium, increased lymph node metastasis both pelvic and aortic, increased extension into the cervix and poorer survival. Apart from the differentiation of the tumour, clear cell, papillary and adenosquamous variants carry a poorer prognosis.

Lymph node involvement and decreasing survival rates correlate well with increasing depths of myometrial invasion.

The pattern of lymph node involvement has recently become more clear. Early studies suggested that the primary lymphatic drainage for endometrial carcinoma was via the tubal and ovarian lymphatics to the para-aortic glands and that pelvic lymph nodes usually only became involved when the cervix was infiltrated by the disease (Stage II). It has become apparent that even in Stage I disease the pelvic nodes may be involved in 11% of patients. Furthermore, in 60% of cases where there is pelvic lymph node involvement the para-aortic glands are also involved. This being so, the choice of the initial operation, i.e. total abdominal hysterectomy and bilateral salpingo-oophorectomy or radical hysterectomy with lymphadenectomy, becomes another variable in the survival of the patient in Stage I disease.

It has not been customary for peritoneal washings to be taken for cytological examination in cases of carcinoma of the endometrium although this is well established in the staging of ovarian carcinoma. Malignant cells in the peritoneum may arise from occult pelvic or abdominal disease or by tubal or lymphatic spread. Positive cytology has been reported in one series in 15% of Stage I disease. The prognosis was poor, half not surviving.

From the information you have given how do you consider such patients should be managed surgically?

The baseline is the current situation. Carcinoma of the endometrium is the commonest female genital tract malignancy. The overall crude 5-year survival rate is in the order of 66% and so it is not in any way a benign condition.

To improve the outcome, variables to be considered include the selection of the primary procedure, the decision to employ pre- or postoperative vaginal radiotherapy or neither of these, and the use of external radiation to pelvic and/or para-aortic glands.

After the staging procedure the extent of the disease will be known in most cases and the nature and differentiation of the cancer will have been established.

No advantage has been demonstrated for the routine use of radiotherapy before or after surgery in Stage I disease. Where the disease is thought to be restricted to the corpus and the disease is a well differentiated adenocarcinoma then a total abdominal hysterectomy and bilateral salpingo-oophorectomy would probably suffice. If the histology demonstrated an aggressive variant or a poorly differentiated carcinoma then a radical procedure would be indicated at the outset. An exception here would be the papillary carcinoma which spreads like ovarian carcinoma primarily to the para-aortic glands beyond the limits of the radical hysterectomy. A total abdominal hysterectomy and bilateral salpingo-oophorectomy would then be appropriate. If, after the radical procedure the glands were involved then external radiation would be required. The purpose of the management is to select those women who are at greatest risk for pelvic lymph node involvement for radical surgery, so that lymph node involvement can be identified and radiotherapy can then be given only to those women who require it. At surgery peritoneal washings should be taken for cytological study.

If the original decision had been to perform a total abdominal hysterectomy and bilateral salpingo-oophorectomy then the operative specimen should be examined. If the penetration of the tumour is more than one-third of the myometrium or if the cervix was found unexpectedly to be involved, lymphadenectomy can then be undertaken. Should the peritoneal cytology subsequently be reported positive following either primary procedure, external radiation to the pelvis and/or para-aortic glands should be considered.

A radical hysterectomy is irrelevant if there is already spread to the para-aortic nodes. If facilities exist for frozen sections of para-aortic gland biopsies then a positive result at operation would avoid unnecessary radical surgery.

Logically Stage II disease should be treated by radical hysterectomy as the disease behaves like Stage Ib carcinoma of the cervix with spread to the parametrium, pelvic lymph nodes and upper vagina. The high incidence of pelvic lymph node involvement in Stage II disease (36%) makes lymphadenopathy an attractive proposition. However it would seem that radical hysterectomy offers no clear advantage in terms of survival than total abdominal hysterectomy and bilateral salpingo-oophorectomy with elective radiation therapy to the pelvis.

Total abdominal hysterectomy and bilateral salpingo-oophorectomy should be attempted either before or after radiation treatment in Stages III and IV. For stage IV disease progestogens and multiple drug chemotherapy can contribute to longevity in these patients.

Discussion

It is clear that the prognosis for endometrial carcinoma is dictated by the extent of the disease at presentation. The staging of the disease by simple clinical examination has led to many ambiguities especially the distinction between Stage I and Stage II. The FIGO Gynaecological Oncology Committee meeting in October 1988 decided that corpus carcinoma should be surgically staged so that additional factors of prognostic importance are included in the staging. This protocol replaces that of 1971 which was based only on the findings at EUA, D and C, i.e. the location of the tumour, the length of the uterine cavity, the histology of the curettings and the detection of extension or metastases by clinical methods.

It should be noted that peritoneal cytology is a component of this staging and therefore should be undertaken in all cases.

Histopathology – the degree of differentiation by Grade (International Society of Gynaecological Pathologists):

G1: 5% or less of a non-squamous or non-morular solid growth pattern.

G2: 6–50% of a non-squamous or non-morular solid growth pattern.

G3: More than 50% of a non-squamous or non-morular solid growth pattern.

The grades G1–G3 are also influenced by the degree of nuclear atypia and the type of tumour.

Staging of tumours:

Stage I		
Ia	G1, 2, 3	Tumour limited to the endometrium
Ib	G1, 2, 3	Invasion $<$ 1/2 of the myometrium
Ic	G1, 2, 3	Invasion $>$ 1/2 of the myometrium
Stage II		
IIA	G1, 2, 3	Endocervical glandular involvement only
IIB	G1, 2, 3	Cervical stromal invasion
Stage III		
IIIA	G1, 2, 3	Tumour extends to serosa and/or adnexa and/or positive peritoneal cytology
IIIB	G1, 2, 3	Metastasis to pelvic and/or para-aortic lymph nodes
Stage IV		
IVA	G1, 2, 3	Tumour invasion of bladder and/or bowel mucosa
IVB	G1, 2, 3	Distant metastases including intra-abdominal and/or inguinal lymph nodes

As this classification is surgical it does not assist in the initial management of the patient. Decisions on the nature of surgery will depend on the considerations discussed in the case presentation above. The earlier staging does not translate into the new protocol and therefore the literature will need to be interpreted with caution in future to ensure that like is being compared with like.

Outcome

The patient was treated by total abdominal hysterectomy and bilateral salpingo-oophorectomy.

The uterus measured 10 cm in length and 5.0 × 4.5 cm at the fundus. The endometrium was 0.5 cm thick and appeared haemorrhagic. In the upper part of the uterus near the right cornu was a firm pale tumour 3.0 × 2.0 cm. Histologically the tumour was a deeply invasive moderate to poorly differentiated endometrial adenocarcinoma. It showed foci of squamous metaplasia. The tumour extended close to the serosa at two points but had not breached the surface. The tubes and ovaries were free of tumour. The cervix was not involved.

This patient recovered well and is free of disease 6 years later.

Comment

It is not impossible for the candidate to be presented with a patient that has already been comprehensively investigated and a diagnosis established. This information may be made available to him. At least this should suggest possible lines of questioning, but the examiner may make an unexpected approach as in this case when he asked the candidate to develop a protocol for management based on data that he has volunteered rather than simply an account of management employed by his seniors.

Further reading

HAMMOND, I. G. (1987) Endometrial carcinoma: is there a place for radical surgery? *Ballieres Clinical Obstetrics and Gynaecology*, **1**, 247–262

SHEPHERD, J. H. (1989) Revised FIGO staging for gynaecological cancer. *British Journal of Obstetrics and Gynaecology*, **96**, 889–892 (Commentary)

Case 23

The patient, a 25-year-old primigravidae married to a lorry driver was referred by her GP to the hospital clinic for booking with a history of 11 weeks amenorrhoea. Her clinical examination was satisfactory. Her blood pressure was recorded as 140/80 mmHg. Urinalysis was normal. She was reviewed 6 weeks later when an ultrasound examination confirmed a singleton pregnancy appropriate to dates. Her blood pressure was 130/80 mmHg. The patient was referred to her GP for shared antenatal care. Her examination at 27 weeks was normal. Urinalysis was clear. Two weeks later she was symptom free, her blood pressure was recorded as 150/110 mmHg and dipstick testing of the urine confirmed albumin ++. Pitting oedema of her ankles was elicited. Her weight gain between weeks 11 and 29 had been 10 kg. She was admitted to hospital.

She is now at 31 weeks gestation. Her BP is 170/105 mmHg. She is symptom free. There is pitting oedema to midshin and over the sacrum. The optic fundi are normal and the tendon reflexes are normal and symmetrical. The uterine size is equivalent to dates; the fundal height is 34 cm. The fetus presents by the breech, it does not feel small and there is adequate liquor present. The fetal heart is heard.

Questions

What is your diagnosis?

Pre-eclampsia. A patient with a normal blood pressure and normal urinalysis in the first trimester has developed hypertension and proteinuria at 29 weeks gestation.

What investigations would you have instituted on her admission to hospital?

The ward staff would be informed that the patient required special observation until instructions are given to the contrary. The junior staff should be briefed as to the potential problems for the case and prompted to pursue the results of investigations should there be delay in reports reaching the ward.

Initially blood pressure recordings should be taken hourly, extending the period between observations to every 4 h when the situation is stable. A fluid input and output chart would be commenced immediately incorporating a cumulative input and output calculation at each recording. Each individual specimen of urine should be collected and tested by dipstick. From the first morning, 24-h collections of urine should be aggregated and submitted for 24-h urinary protein estimation. The same sample can be used in conjunction with a serum creatinine for a calculation of the renal creatinine clearance.

Blood samples should be taken daily for haemoglobin, haematocrit and platelet count and for urea, creatinine and electrolyte estimations. Blood for urate and liver enzymes will be taken on alternate days together with samples for a clotting screen and the detection of fibrin degradation products.

A comprehensive ultrasound examination is indicated to exclude signs of IUGR, unsuspected fetal abnormality and to provide a baseline biophysical profile.

The fetal well-being should be ascertained by fetal movement counting, daily unstressed cardiotocography, and a weekly assessment of the biophysical profile together with serial measurement of the biparietal diameter, head circumference, and abdominal circumference.

What therapy if any would you prescribe?

The patient is symptom free. She has been in hospital for 2 weeks and her blood pressure is stable with a diastolic value of 105 mmHg. If the blood pressure were to rise, then one might entertain the possibility of hypotensive agents, although at this gestation and with neonatal facilities available deterioration of the maternal state might be better dealt with by delivery of the fetus.

These are the results of tests taken on the day the patient was admitted. Have you any comments?

Haemoglobin:		12.8 g/dl
Hct ratio:		0.380
Platelets:		225×10^9/l
Urea	(2.5–7.0 mmol/l):	5.2 mmol/l
Creatinine	(45–120 μmol/l):	77.0 μmol/l
Urate	(0.20–0.40 mmol/l):	0.40 mmol/l
Albumin	(38–47 g/l):	31.0 g/l
Total protein	(60–80 g/l):	59.0 g/l
AST	(15–34 IU/l):	25.0 IU/l
Alkaline phosphatase	(60–130 IU/l):	200.0 IU/l
Gamma-GT	(10–30 IU/l):	28.0 IU/l
PT	(14–18 s):	14.0 s
PPT	(36–48 s):	37.0 s
FDPs	(2–8 ug/ml):	< 10 ug/ml
Urinary protein/24 h:		5.7 g/l
Creatinine clearance:		80 ml/min

The results are entered on a standard laboratory form. The normal values quoted relate to the non-pregnant state.

There is no evidence of disseminated intravascular coagulation. The platelet count is normal, there is no rise in circulating fibrin degradation products, and the clotting screen is normal.

There is very heavy and pathological proteinuria. There is a natural fall in the total plasma proteins and albumin in pregnancy in the order of 10 g per litre. The falls recorded therefore are consistent with the pregnant state. The alkaline phosphatase level is raised reflecting placental production of this enzyme. The hepatocellular enzymes remain normal in pregnancy and no disturbance has been demonstrated.

The glomerular filtration rate is characteristically increased in pregnancy. In the third trimester the creatinine clearance should be in the order of 130 ml/min. The value of 80 ml/min suggests impairment of renal function if the urinary collection was complete.

Although the plasma levels of creatinine, urea and urate are normal for the non-pregnant state they are significantly raised for pregnancy confirming a degree of renal impairment.

We have listed the patient's results to the present. Have you any observations to make?

Day	3	5	7	9	11	13
BP (mmHg)	180/105	170/100	180/100	170/105	180/110	170/105
Hb (g/dl)	11.9	12.2	12.3	12.6	12.5	12.8
Platelets ($\times 10^9$/l)	180	190	186	195	208	210
Hct	0.380	0.350	0.355	0.384	0.378	0.380
Urea (mmol/l)	5.8	6.3	5.8	5.8	6.9	7.6
Creat (μmol/l)	81	84	83	89	89	93
Urate (mmol/l)	0.37	0.40	0.46	0.48	–	0.52
AST (IU/l)	28	28	29	32	38	42
Gamma-GT (IU/l)	33	–	38	40	42	42
C-Clear (ml/min)	86	–	75	–	–	68
U-protein (g/24-h)	6.0	–	5.8	–	–	6.8

The results reveal a falling creatinine clearance rate associated with significant elevation of the plasma urate, urea and creatinine. The blood pressure is showing no particular trend upwards and there is no suggestion yet of DIC developing, at least in terms of the platelet count. There is a rise in the levels of liver enzymes suggesting involvement of that organ. Delivery should not be delayed much longer.

What are the symptoms of impending eclampsia?

There may be none. Nausea or sickness is significant in a patient with pre-eclampsia. Epigastric pain, headache, visual disturbances and hyper-reflexia are more immediate prodromal symptoms.

If this patient's blood pressure were to rise and the patient to have an eclamptic fit, what would you do?

The immediate requirement is to establish that the airway is intact and prevent a further convulsion. The convulsion should be controlled by the administration of diazepam 5–10 mg i.v. or more if required. Hydralazine 20 mg is given as a bolus followed by 5 mg every 20 min until the diastolic BP is 100–110 mmHg.

With the onset of eclampsia conservation of the pregnancy further is inappropriate. The maternal condition will only be reversed by the delivery of the baby. Assuming the baby is still alive following the fit, at this gestation and with the breech presenting the delivery should be by caesarean section.

With the history of an eclamptic fit or in the presence of deteriorating severe pre-eclampsia it is essential to avoid subsequent fits. The patient requires intensive care facilities on the labour ward, certainly for 24 h after delivery and special nursing for a further 24 h, until such time as the blood pressure is controlled and normal renal function has been confirmed.

Once the immediate emergency has been controlled an intravenous line is established with Hartmans solution and the patient catheterized. The catheter should be connected to a receiver graduated to permit the hourly measurement of the urinary output.

The aim of management is to:
Control the blood pressure.
Prevent eclampsia.
Provide adequate analgesia.
Safeguard renal function.
Coordinate the fluid balance and to avoid circulatory overload.

The maternal condition should be monitored by continuous ECG, and automated recording of the BP at 15 m intervals. The fluid input and output should be recorded hourly and a running cumulative total calculated. Specimens of urine should be tested for protein and blood and the urine osmololality determined 12-hourly or in the presence of oliguria. Every 6 h blood should be taken for haemoglobin, haematocrit, platelet and electrolyte estimation. At the same intervals a clotting screen and measurement of fibrin degradation products should be performed. This protocol is not rigid and tests may be done more frequently if the clinical picture suggests it.

Control of blood pressure Women with severe pre-eclampsia are hypovolaemic. Volume expansion with hyperosmolar solutions improves the haemoconcentration and output of urine as well as lowering the mean arterial pressure (MAP). (MAP = systolic BP + 2 × diastolic BP per/3 mmHg)

The 400 ml of plasma protein fraction are administered through the intravenous line. If the MAP is subsequently < 125 mmHg, Hartman's solution is used to maintain the line (1000 ml every 12 h). If the hourly urinary output falls below 0.5 ml/kg per h then a central venous line is inserted to detect any tendency to circulatory overload.

If the MAP remains above 125 mmHg, despite the use of bolus injections of hydralazine then the drug should be given by syringe pump at the rate of 5–10 mg/h. Should this fail to modify the blood pressure or the patient develops a tachycardia labetalol can be given at the rate of 5 mg/min until the MAP falls below 125 mmHg and the pulse remains below 100 beats/min.

Prevention of fits After the control of the fit with diazepam, phenytoin sodium is given i.v. by syringe pump. The loading dose is 10 mg/kg given at a rate of 25 mg /min. Two hours later the plasma phenytoin level is estimated and loading completed by the administration of a dose of 7.5 mg/kg given as before. Plasma phenytoin levels are measured 6-hourly. The aim is to keep the plasma level in the therapeutic range of 10–20 mg/l if necessary by giving 250 mg of the drug 6 h after the end of the loading infusion. The drug can have toxic side-effects producing cardiac arrhythmia, drowsiness, nausea, nystagmus, diplopia and ataxia; consequently, if the plasma level 6 h after loading is in excess of 12 mg/l the maintenance dose is withheld. If the patient is undelivered 12 h after loading the 500 mg is given i.v. but if delivered and taking by mouth, oral maintenance therapy of 250 mg 12-hourly for 3 days is started.

Optimal *pain relief* is given by epidural anaesthesia. If the plan is to induce labour then the colloid challenge at the start is sufficient to preload the patient. In such hypovolaemic patients the administration of an epidural anaesthetic can seriously compromise the placental circulation. If the plan is to deliver the patient by caesarean section immediately the patient is stabilized, then additional preloading with 400 ml Hartman's solution is indicated.

In the event of oliguria developing (< 0.5ml/kg per h) then a CVP line is inserted . If the CVP is normal or low then a colloid challenge with 100 ml PPF is justified. This may improve the renal function by correcting any hypovolaemia. If the CVP is raised or rises following a colloid challenge then the patient is not hypovolaemic and renal failure is a possibility.

You have described a complicated regimen using a potentially toxic drug. Why not use a more conventional agent to prevent convulsions such as chlormethiazole or diazepam?

The regimen is complicated but it is designed to achieve the aims stated and to avoid iatrogenic complications. The maternal mortality report of 1982–1984 recorded maternal deaths in one pre-eclamptic and two eclamptic patients as a result of fluid overload.

The alternative agents you stipulate are not without their side-effects. Chlormethiazole is only anticonvulsant at doses which are sedative to both mother and fetus. Fear of excessive maternal sedation often leads to inadequate anticonvulsant therapy. The use of the usual 0.8% solution entails the infusion of relatively large volumes of crystalloid fluid (500 ml 6–8-hourly). As prophylaxis must be continued for a minimum of 24 h after delivery this can lead to fluid overload. Diazepam has a wide safety margin for the mother but there is a real risk of neonatal hypotonus, respiratory depression and hypothermia. Furthermore the neonate, especially if preterm, is unable to metabolize or excrete diazepam or its active metabolite desmethyldiazepam adequately so that the adverse effects may be very prolonged and on occasion exchange transfusion may be required. Phenytoin is an effective anticonvulsant without being a sedative and the patient remains awake and cooperative throughout. It is given as a small volume infusion and has been shown to have an independent hypotensive effect.

Discussion

With pulmonary embolism, hypertensive diseases of pregnancy are the commonest cause of maternal death in the UK. The commonest causes of death are intracranial haemorrhage, cerebral oedema, hepatic and/or renal failure, cardiac failure and coagulation complications. Deaths from pulmonary oedema secondary to fluid overload during the management of severe cases have been recorded. The hypertensive disorders also are an important cause of fetal loss and morbidity. The perinatal mortality associated with chronic hypertension and pregnancy induced hypertension is similar to the equivalent normotensive patient. If pre-eclampsia becomes superimposed upon existing chronic hypertension then the perinatal loss is doubled. Pre-eclampsia increases the perinatal mortality largely because of IUGR, abruption and preterm delivery in the interest of the mother.

The terminology surrounding these conditions has been confused but the International Society for the Study of Hypertension in Pregnancy has recommended the classification (1988) shown:

DEFINITIONS

Hypertension	1.	One measurement of diastolic blood pressure of 110 mmHg or more, or
	2.	Two consecutive measurements of diastolic blood pressure of 90 mmHg or more, 4 h or more apart
Proteinuria	1.	Total protein excretion of 300 mg or more per 24 h
	2.	+++ (1 g/l) or more on a reagent strip if the SG is more than 1030 or, + (0.3 g/l) or more if the SG is less than 1030

CLASSIFICATION

Gestational hypertension or proteinuria	Hypertension or proteinuria developing after 20 weeks of pregnancy in a previously normotensive non-proteinuric woman
Gestational proteinuric hypertension (pre-eclampsia)	Hypertension in combination with proteinuria developing after 20 weeks gestation in a previously normotensive non-proteinuric woman
Chronic hypertension or renal disease	Hypertension and/or proteinuria in a woman with chronic hypertension or chronic renal disease diagnosed before, during or persisting after pregnancy
Chronic hypertension with superimposed pre-eclampsia	Proteinuria developing for the first time during pregnancy in a woman with chronic hypertension
Unclassified hypertension and/or proteinuria	Hypertension and/or proteinuria found at the first antenatal visit after 20 weeks gestation
Eclampsia	The occurrence of generalized convulsions during pregnancy, labour or within 7 days of delivery, and not caused by epilepsy or other convulsive disorders

The blood pressure should be taken with a standard sphygmomanometer the diastolic value being read at the 'muffling' of the sounds (Korotkoff phase 4). The cuff should be at the level of the atrium. Note that oedema, overall weight gain, and incremental weight gain no longer contribute to the diagnosis of pre-eclampsia.

The usual pattern of antenatal care is designed to pick up the onset of gestational hypertension or pre-eclampsia when they are most likely to develop in the last trimester. There are consumer and professional requests to reduce the number of antenatal visits in early and mid-pregnancy. However, although routine antenatal screening for hypertensive disorders before 28 weeks may yield but few cases they are crucial because these are the cases that contribute predominately to the maternal and fetal morbidity and mortality associated with these disorders.

Proteinuria is a late sign of renal involvement in pre-eclampsia. An earlier change is a reduced uric acid clearance resulting in a rise in plasma urate. This change is caused by tubular malfunction and precedes the impairment of glomerular filtration when proteinuria develops and there is a rise in the plasma creatinine and urea. An elevated plasma urate in the presence of gestational hypertension predicts the onset of pre-eclampsia. Women with chronic hypertension have normal urate levels. The mean plasma urate levels in the second and third trimester are 214 µmol/l and 269 µmol/l respectively. Concentrations over 350 µmol/l indicate significant pre-eclampsia and are associated with a high perinatal mortality particularly between 28 and 36 weeks gestation. Plasma urea concentrations of 6 mmol/l and creatinine concentrations of 90 µmol/l are significantly raised for pregnancy. In the normal event, the glomerular filtration rate is raised in pregnancy. In the last trimester, a creatinine clearance of 119 ml/min represents the 5th centile of a normal population. Regular estimations of these values is an integral part of the management of pre-eclampsia.

The liver is also a target organ in pre-eclampsia and often forgotten. The Maternal Mortality Report draws attention to the to the lack of symptoms even when this organ is severely involved. Liver damage is particularly associated with DIC in pre-eclampsia. Microangiopathic haemolysis may develop.

The repeated measurement of blood urea, creatinine, urate, platelets and liver enzymes are essential to provide an early indication of organ involvement.

There is clearly a relationship between gestational hypertension and the subsequent development of pre-eclampsia. It is not inevitable. For women who become hypertensive before 33 weeks 31% of nulliparae and 21% of multiparae will develop pre-eclampsia. For those who become hypertensive after 33 weeks gestation only 6 and 10% respectively will develop proteinuria.

Gestational hypertension carries little risk to mother or fetus unless proteinuria supervenes. Consequently a variety of pharmacological agents have been introduced usually at an arbitrary blood pressure value to prevent this transition or to delay its onset.

Methyldopa, labetalol and atenolol seem to succeed in preventing the escalation of pregnancy-induced hypertension but there is no convincing evidence that this therapy prevents the development of proteinuria or improves the perinatal mortality. The aim of therapy is to keep the maternal blood pressure below 170/110 mmHg to avoid the complications of hypertension *per se*.

Pre-eclampsia remains the enigma of obstetric practice.

Patterns of antenatal care have been established to identify the condition as soon as it develops because of its unpredictable and sometimes fulminating progression with severe consequences for mother and baby. It is responsible for the incarceration within hospital of large numbers of otherwise healthy pregnant women for often long periods of time. Contrarily, some patients are admitted only to be discharged soon after, as the diagnosis made in the clinic fails to establish. The dislocation of family life is enormous. The distinction made between pregnancy-induced (gestational) hypertension with the emphasis on out-patient management, and pre-eclampsia (proteinuric) hypertension has gone some way to relieve the situation, but there remain the few who progress rapidly from the one category to the other. The use of plasma urate estimations to identify those who will progress is an attractive proposition but there has been no blind clinical trial to determine the efficacy of this management in terms of eventual outcome.

A resolution of the problem could be the introduction of a therapy that would prevent the development of the condition safely in all women. Established pre-eclampsia is associated with a coagulopathy characterized by a consumption of factor VIII, increased levels of fibrin degradation products and reduced circulating platelets. Aspirin inhibits the enzyme cyclo-oxygenase in platelets preventing the synthesis of the platelet aggregating agent thromboxane A2. The drug is widely used therefore for prophylaxis following cases of myocardial infarction, cerebral ischaemia and coronary bypass. In pregnancy, two trials have suggested that low dose asprin may at least delay the rate of progression of the disease, reducing the perinatal mortality by reducing the number of very preterm deliveries. Many hospitals in the UK are involved in the CLASP trial (Collaborative Low-dose Aspirin Study in Pregnancy) to ascertain the efficacy of low dose aspirin (60 mg/day) in high risk pregnancies to prevent or modify the development of pre-eclampsia and IUGR.

Comment

On being asked the management of such a case the candidate should be able to respond, even with a complicated protocol, without hesitation. At this level such systems of management should be automatically recalled but nevertheless applied with comprehension and understanding.

In answering the question about investigations to be performed in this case no mention was made of the reasons for the investigations selected. The candidate is answering the question posed. If the examiner wants further explanation he will ask for it subsequently or interrupt during the answer.

The protocol for the management of eclampsia described is not in common use, but it would be the schedule used by the registrars in the unit concerned and with which they would be familiar. The important thing is for candidates to understand the rationale for the regimens they employ and to be aware of any risks. They should also know of other alternatives and their limitations. It is always wiser in the long run to speak from personal experience rather than try to anticipate what the examiner might like to hear.

Further reading

BEAUFILS, M., UZAN, S., DONSIMONI, R. and COLAU, J. C. (1985) Prevention of pre-eclampsia by early antiplatelet therapy. *Lancet*, **i**, 840–842

DAVEY, D. A. and MacGILLIVRAY, I. (1988) The classification and definition of the hypertensive disorders of pregnancy. *American Journal of Obstetrics and Gynecology*, **158**, 892–898

MOOSA, S. M. and EL ZAYAT, S. G. (1987) Phenytoin solution in severe pre-eclampsia. *Lancet*, **i**, 1417–1420

REDMAN, C. W. G., WILLIAMS, G. F., JONES, D. D. and WILKINSON, R. H. (1977) Plasma urate and serum deoxycytidylate deaminase measurements for the early diagnosis of pre-eclampsia. *British Journal of Obstetrics and Gynaecology*, **84**, 904–908

RUBIN, P. C., BUTTERS, L., CLARK, D. M., REYNOLDS, B., SUMNER, D. J., STEEDMAN, D., LOW, R. A. and REID, J. L. (1983) Placebo controlled trial of atenolol in treatment of pregnancy associated hypertension. *Lancet*, **i**, 431–434

WALLENBERG, H. C. S. (1988) Hemodynamics in hypertensive pregnancy. In *Hypertension in Pregnancy* (eds W. H. Birkenhoger and J. L. Reid). *Handbook of Hypertension*, Vol. 10 (ed. P. C. Rubin), Elsevier, Amsterdam, pp. 66–102

Case 24

The 17-year-old patient was referred to the gynaecological clinic by her GP because of primary amenorrhoea. She was the only child of a couple who had married late in life. The mother had been 40 years of age at the time of conception. For religious reasons the couple had declined amniocentesis in pregnancy. The pregnancy had been normal and the baby weighed 3725 g at birth. She had achieved her milestones for walking and talking at the expected times. Mother and father were of normal stature. The mother was 168 cm tall and the father 179 cm tall. The patient had left school at 16 years of age without any qualifications. She was currently attending a youth training scheme for basic office work. She lived at home with her parents and had few interests apart from taking part in the various activities at her local church. She was generally happy and was enjoying her work. She took a full diet and there was no history of dieting. She complained of no abdominal pain and was taking no drugs. Her mother had menstruated at 13 years of age.

On examination she was of short stature (150 cm tall) and weighed 45 kg. The proportions of her limbs to her body appeared normal. The facies appeared normal with a normal hair line. There was no goitre and she was clinically euthyroid. Breast development was completely absent as was axillary hair. The chest and trunk were rather stocky. A small amount of pubic hair was present. Her blood pressure was 110/60 mmHg with normal peripheral pulses. The external genitalia were infantile. A pelvic examination was not attempted but a rectal examination suggested the presence of a vagina and a small uterus.

Questions

How would you summarize this case?

The diagnosis is of primary amenorrhoea in a young woman of short stature and absent or minimal secondary sexual development.

Could this be constitutional, the girl being a late developer?

This is unlikely. The mother menstruated at a normal age and if the problem were merely late development there would have been some secondary sexual development by this chronological age. As the secondary sexual development is absent then it suggests an endocrine cause for the amenorrhoea rather than cryptorchidism.

What endocrine disturbance you have in mind?

Either pituitary or ovarian failure, i.e. gonadal dysgenesis. Had there been good breast development in association with absent or very scant pubic hair then androgen insensitivity (testicular feminization) would be a possibility but those patients are usually of normal stature.

What investigations would you undertake?

The diagnosis should be established by a chromosomal analysis and an estimation of the serum gonadotrophin levels.

The results of the initial investigations are detailed below. What do they show?

LH:	30 U/l
FSH:	> 40 U/l
17-beta-oestradiol:	40 pmol/l
Progesterone:	< 4 nmol/l
Prolactin:	320 mU/l
T4:	120 nmol/l
TSH:	4 mU/l
Random blood sugar:	3.5 mmol/l
GTT:	Normal
Leucocyte culture karyotype:	46XX/45XO (60%/40%) Mosaic
Lateral skull X-ray:	Normal

The gonadotrophin levels are raised indicating gonadal failure or at least the absence of any oestrogenic inhibition. Consequently the oestrogen level is low and progesterone is below the limit of the assay. She is euthyroid and her glucose tolerance is unimpaired. Her prolactin level is normal. The karyotype confirms a mosaic pattern 46XX/45XO. The picture is consistent with gonadal dysgenesis the abnormal cell line XO involving the gonad.

By gonadal dysgenesis do you mean Turner's syndrome?

No, the eponym 'Turner's syndrome' is best reserved for that manifestation of gonadal dysgenesis associated with a 45XO karyotype. The facies are distinctive with a low hair line, prominent epicanthic folds, a small mouth and micrognatha and low set ears which may be deformed. The neck is short and wide and may be webbed. Breast development is absent and the nipples are widely spaced. The trunk is broad and shapeless. There is cubitus valgus. Deformities of the wrists, fingers and toes can occur. Axillary hair is absent and pubic hair is, if present, sparse. Cardiac abnormalities, coarctation of the aorta, renal abnormalities, colour blindness and multiple skin naevi are associated with this condition. Diabetes mellitus and autoimmune thyroid disease are more common in these patients than in the population at large. Patients of short stature and who show only some of the somatic features of Turner's syndrome are best referred to by the term 'Turner's phenotype'.

Would you undertake any further investigations?

I would perform a laparoscopy to establish the presence and configuration of the pelvic organs. Biopsy of the streak ovaries would positively exclude the presence of primary follicles. An IVU is indicated to exclude renal tract anomalies that are common in these patients.

How would you treat this patient?

This patient has presented rather late. Ideally treatment should be commenced about 15 years of age. Breast development and menstruation can be promoted by the taking of hormones. A low dose combined oral contraceptive can be given from the outset. However, cyclical oestrogen first of all in low doses (ethinyloestradiol 10 μg once daily for 3 of 4 weeks for 3–6 months) and then high doses (ethinyloestradiol 20 μg for 3 of 4 weeks for 3–6 months) have been advocated initially, before supplementing the higher dose regimen with norethisterone 5 mg daily on days 12–21 after a year. In the long-term management a progestational component is essential to avoid endometrial hyperplasia and in some patients the induction of endometrial carcinoma.

Equally important from the patient's point of view is the careful and sensitive counselling that is necessary as the diagnosis unfolds and the implications for the future are recognized. In particular she will have to cope with the recognition of her infertility.

What other chromosomal abnormalities may be associated with gonadal dysgenesis?

Almost all are variants of 'Turner mosaicism'. XO/XY, XO/XXY, XO/XX/XXX and XO/XY/XYYY are described. There is a group of individuals with gonadal dysgenesis who, apart from sexual infantilism manifest none of the stigmata associated with Turner's syndrome or Turner's phenotypes. The chromosomal complement may be 46XY or 46XX. As there are no gonads these individuals will all be phenotypically female. This group are referred to as cases of 'pure gonadal dysgenesis'.

Would you treat these Turner phenotypes in the same way as the case you have presented?

If the karyotype has a Y chromosome in its constitution there is a one in three chance of gonadal malignancy, either a gonadoblastoma or a dysgerminoma. In these cases the streak gonads should be removed as soon as the karyotype is defined.

Discussion

Patients with classical Turner's syndrome are deficient in chromosomal material. The evidence is that the genes that protect against the stigmata of Turner's syndrome are carried on the short arms of the two sex chromosomes, XX or XY. Those which protect against streak gonads and which are responsible for gonadal development are on the long arms. It is the loss of genetic material essential for gonadal development that results in absent secondary sexual development and primary amenorrhoea. The loss of further genetic material on the short arm of the same X chromosome produces the stigmata of the disease. The degree of expression depends upon the locus and the amount of the material lost to produce such signs as short stature, webbing, short metatarsals, coarctation of the aorta etc. The complete syndrome develops therefore when there is only a solitary X sex chromosome (45XO). Deletions from the short arm of one X chromosome (46 XXp−) or again the absence of a short arm with a long arm isochromosome (46XXqi) can produce the phenotype. There may be mosaicism with such cell lines contributing but if the abnormal cell line affects only non-gonadal tissue Turner's stigmata may be present without gonadal dysgenesis and the hormonal sequelae.

When there is a mosaic or an abnormal X chromosome rather than an absent X or Y chromosome the expression of the Turner's phenotype can be very variable. The picture is influenced by the proportion of normal to abnormal cells and their distribution in the embryo. If a significant proportion of normal 46 XX cells inherit the genital ridge then some ovarian differentiation may occur at puberty with a degree of secondary sexual development and even menstruation.

It follows that the prognosis attributed to a particular case in the mosaic situation cannot be established until after the age of puberty because a few patients will achieve menstruation and a very few conceive. If the chromosomal picture is unequivocal and the gonadotrophin levels achieve menopausal levels then gonadal dysgenesis is virtually assured. If there are discordant features to suggest possible ovarian activity, e.g. some breast development, then ovarian biopsy to identify primordial follicles or a gonadotrophic challenge to the ovary to produce an oestrogen response will clarify the situation.

Outcome

The patient was treated according to the regimen described. Breast development occurred to the patient's delight and menstruation was achieved. It had been considered before her presentation that she had been a well-adjusted and content individual. It was apparent after treatment that her life had been transformed. She had developed a new confidence, secured full-time employment and was returning to adult education to get some qualifications.

Comment

Cases of gonadal dysgenesis have been presented to candidates in the examination. In such cases a pelvic examination can be inappropriate. The examiner will concentrate rather on the history and the candidate's evaluation of the problem. The clinical examination result depends upon the candidate's performance in both the obstetric and the gynaecological case. It is the demonstration of overall clinical competence that is being tested.

Further reading

DEWHURST, C. J. (1971) Sex chromosome abnormalities and the gynaecologist. *British Journal of Obstetrics and Gynaecology*, **78**, 1058–1076

Case 25

The patient is 31 years old and in her fifth pregnancy. She lives with the unemployed father of her last two children and her last child in a council house. Her other children have been adopted. She receives supplementary benefit. She has been asthmatic since a child and attends a chest clinic under consultant supervision. She has had numerous admissions to hospital for acute exacerbations of the asthma,twice in the year preceding the current pregnancy. Four years after her last pregnancy she developed insulin dependent diabetes (White classification group B).

The pregnancy was planned. She had received depot Provera for contraception since her last pregnancy and this was discontinued 18 months ago. The menstrual cycle had established itself regularly, 4–7/28–30. The LMP was on 17 April and specifically recorded. She is now 36 weeks pregnant.

In 1979 she was delivered at term by midcavity forceps of a female infant weighing 3430 g. The indication for forceps was delay in the second stage. A year later she was delivered spontaneously of a male infant weighing 3232 g at 38 weeks gestation The pregnancy had been uncomplicated. This child subsequently developed hydrocephalus secondary to a congenital Dandy Walker cyst. A ventriculoperitoneal shunt was inserted. The child suffers from grand mal seizures and is mentally retarded. The third pregnancy in 1982 was normal, with the spontaneous delivery at term of a male infant weighing 3629 g. The last pregnancy in 1983 ended with the spontaneous delivery at 38 weeks of a female infant weighing 3510 g.The pregnancy was interrupted by several admissions for the exacerbation of her asthma.

She neither smokes nor takes alcohol. There is no significant family history. She is allergic to eggs which precipitate a generalized rash but there is no history of allergy to drugs.

She booked at the antenatal clinic with a history of 7 weeks amenorrhoea. An ultrasound examination was performed which confirmed an intrauterine pregnancy with a crown-rump length of 18 mm. She was normotensive and urinalysis was negative. Her examination was normal apart from her weight (91 kg), and an expiratory wheeze consistent with her history of asthma. Her medication was as follows:

Insulin 07.30 hours:	Actrapid 5 units/Monotard 5 units
17.30 hours:	Actrapid 10 units/Monotard 8 units
Prednisolone	5 mg twice daily

Salbutamol (Rotacaps®)	400 μg 4 times daily
Beclomethasone (Becloforte®)	500 μg twice daily (two puffs twice daily)
Nedocromil sodium (Tilade®)	4 mgm 4 times daily (two puffs 4 times daily)
Beclomethasone (Beconase®)	50 μg twice daily (two puffs twice daily – nasal)
Salbutamol	8 mg at night

At the booking clinic a random blood glucose level was 4.0 mmol/l. The glycosylated haemoglobin was 5.7%.

She was referred to an obstetric/medical clinic supervised by a consultant obstetrician and a consultant physician in attendance at the same time. For the 24 h before each appointment the patient was instructed to take blood by an automatic stylet before lunch, before tea, before bed, and before breakfast on the morning of the clinic. The patient handed in the samples at the hospital laboratory before progressing to the clinic. The laboratory took a random sample at that time. The results were telephoned to the clinic to be available when the patient was seen.

At 8 weeks the results were: RBS: 5.3 mmol/l, Blood sugar series: 12.00 hours, 5.1 mmol/l; 17.30 hours, 5.8 mmol/l; 21.00 hours, 4.3 mmol/l; 07.00 hours (fasting blood sugar), 3.2 mmol/l.

She felt basically well at this time apart from breathlessness on waking up in the morning. She was placed on a diet of 140 g carbohydrate per day. It was allocated as 30 g for breakfast, 40 g for lunch and 30 g for tea, with 10 g options for a morning and afternoon break and 20 g for a snack before retiring.

It was explained that she should attend the combined clinic weekly. The patient was asked to take fasting and preprandial capillary blood samples by stylet daily and to test these with BM (Bohringer Mannheim) stix. Her readings were logged and reviewed at the weekly visits. The same drops of blood used for the laboratory series each week were also tested on collection by the patient with BM stix. Her results were compared with the laboratory results so that her reliability in reading the BM stix could be assessed. The aim of the clinic was to keep the blood sugar level between 5.0 mmol/l and 7.0 mmol/l.

Although not the normal practice in diabetic cases it was planned that she should be admitted at 30 weeks to stay in hospital, because of the coexistent problem with her asthma and the use of prophylactic steroids.

The asthma proved to be a major problem. She was admitted to hospital for a week at 16 weeks gestation because of an exacerbation of asthma associated with an upper respiratory tract infection. At 20 weeks she spent 2 weeks in hospital with a chest infection which resolved on antibiotics. On each admission as her steroid dosage was increased so did her insulin requirement. A second chest infection coincided with her planned admission at 30 weeks gestation and to relieve bronchospasm her prednisolone was increased to 40 mg/day. Erythromycin was prescribed for the chest infection and subsequently her prednisolone was reduced to 20 mg/day which is her current dose. For the first 48 h s.c. insulin was discontinued and a glucose/insulin/KCl drip instituted. During her stay in hospital she has received her insulin in divided doses at 07.30 hours and 17.30 hours. She daily tests and records her blood sugar with BM stix at 07.00 hours (FBS), 12.00, 15.00, 18.00 and 21.00 hours. She measures her peak expiratory flow rate 6-hourly before and after medication. She has remained on the 140 g carbohydrate diet.

She is now 36 weeks pregnant. She still complains of breathlessness first thing in the morning but is otherwise symptom free. She weighs 107 kg. On examination it is difficult to define much on palpation because of her obesity. It is impossible to be sure whether the uterine size is compatible with dates. A fetus occupies a longitudinal lie with the head palpable three-fifths above the pelvic brim. There is no obvious hydramnios. Her medication is as at booking except that she is taking prednisolone 20 mg/day, her inhalation has been supplemented by ipratropium bromide (Atrovent) 40 μg 4 times daily (2 puffs) and her insulin dosage has increased: 07.30 hours, Actrapid 20 units/Monotard 30 units; 17.30 hours, Actrapid 36 units/Monotard 26 units.

Questions

What are the principal features of this history?

From the patient's point of view her main complaint is her asthma. This is exacerbated with respiratory tract infection. Problems with the chest caused the admissions to hospital. She is taking steroids in oral and in inhaled form and although the latter will not be responsible for significant increases in the blood levels, on the occasions when the oral prescription has been increased there has been a change in her insulin requirement. The situation became so unstable at one point that the situation warranted intravenous insulin infusion.

Apart from the acute fluctuations there has been a gradual increase in the insulin requirement through pregnancy but this is a usual observation. The situation at the onset of the pregnancy was stable. The glycosylated haemoglobin of 5.7% would suggest that control had been adequate over the period of conception and a RBS at booking was within normal limits.

The picture is of a stable insulin-dependent diabetic with problematical asthma, treatment of which interferes with the control of the diabetes.

Her diabetes was well controlled. Apart from the instability at the start of each hospital admission her blood glucose levels remained within the required limits. The lowest value recorded was 2.7 mmol/l and the highest 9.1 mmol/l. These were single readings. As you describe, there was an increase in the insulin requirement overall but this was the cumulation of very slight adjustments as the pregnancy progressed rather than the product of abrupt changes. Her HbA1 levels at 16, 28, 32 and 36 weeks were 4.8, 5.0, 5.2 and 5.2% respectively. What do these results suggest?

The results are within normal limits and would confirm good control of the diabetes. Raised levels would have suggested prolonged episodes of hyperglycaemia. Hypoglycaemic episodes are detrimental to the fetus and these would not be reflected in such results. Hence blood sugar series remain the optimum for monitoring the diabetic in pregnancy.

Comment on her peak expiratory flow measurements.

Peak expiratory flow (ml)	06.00	10.00	14.00	18.00	22.00	06.00	10.00	14.00	18.00	22.00	06.00	10.00
Before bronchodilator	110	250	350	–	300	100	250	350	325	340	150	250
After bronchodilator	170	300	350	–	350	200	300	375	370	400	200	350

Breathlessness is a feature of pregnancy but this patient complained specifically of shortness of breath in the morning. This had been a problem before pregnancy and was no worse during pregnancy. Her peak expiratory flow is markedly reduced in the morning but is improved by the inhalation of bronchodilators. Some improvement occurs whenever bronchodilators are used although the difference is variable, i.e. 25–100 ml. The dips in peak flow at night or in the early morning are characteristic of asthma.

You have described at length her medical management. What other considerations are important?

The assessment of the fetus. Congenital abnormality is commoner in diabetic pregnancies particularly neural tube and cardiac anomalies. The hydrocephalus associated with a Dandy Walker cyst in her second child does not fall into the categories of neural tube defect that tend to recur in subsequent pregnancies. The first ultrasound examination at 7 weeks confirmed the gestational age but was too early to exclude fetal abnormalities. Maternal serum screening at 16 weeks for alpha-fetoprotein and HCG could indicate any increased risk for open neural tube defect or Down's syndrome. Detailed ultrasound examination to exclude fetal abnormality including echocardiography to detect fetal heart anomalies is most likely to be successful if performed around the 18th week. In the presence of insulin-dependent diabetes 30% of infants have cardiomegaly and in 10% there is evidence of cardiac malfunction. Serial ultrasound every 4 weeks thereafter is important to confirm normal fetal growth and to pick up signs of macrosomia, e.g. by measuring disproportionately large abdominal girth. In this case the images may be poor because of the maternal obesity but they should be sufficient to identify the presentation and to exclude hydramnios. From the 36th week ultrasound should be performed weekly and include some form of biophysical profile scoring.

Fetal movement recording should be instituted from 30 weeks and supplemented with daily CTG recording.

The patient with diabetes is more likely to develop pre-eclampsia and the blood pressure should be measured twice daily. For the same reason regular estimation of the plasma urate should be performed. The kidney is a vulnerable organ in the diabetic. The creatinine clearance should be estimated every 4 weeks together with the measurement of the plasma urea and electrolytes.

Apart from the diabetes and asthma, what other features of the history and examination cause you concern?

The social circumstances are not ideal. Four of her previous children are in care and she is in need of financial support.

Apparently the services of a medical social worker were offered at the booking visit but were refused.

This patient is extremely obese. Palpation is difficult and cannot be considered to be adequate. In such cases extremes of fetal weight are even more likely than normal to be missed. Malpresentation may remain unsuspected with the corresponding fear of cord prolapse should the membranes rupture. Correction of a malpresentation by version is unlikely to be successful and probably contraindicated for fear of exerting too much force to achieve an effect. Even simple procedures such as recording the blood pressure become less reproducible in such patients even when a suitable cuff is employed. Nevertheless, there is probably a true association between obesity and pre-eclampsia. Any tendency to dyspnoea will be aggravated. In the event of a general anaesthetic being required intubation may prove difficult with the risk of anoxia in the fetus. The siting of epidural anaesthetics may prove impossible. Caesarean section is technically more difficult in such patients both from the point of view of access and the tying of knots when the suture material and gloves are slippery with fat. After surgery, chest infections are more likely because of reduced ventilation and there is the increased risk of deep vein thrombosis. Even without surgery this risk is increased. Wounds are less likely to heal by first intention. Postpartum haemorrhage is more common and the patient's veins are less accessible for infusion.

Her high parity places her at greater risk for all forms of antepartum haemorrhage, anaemia, hypertensive disease, malpresentation, 'multip disproportion', dysfunctional and precipitate labour, postpartum haemorrhage and uterine rupture.

When would you deliver this patient?

This patient's diabetes has been well controlled probably from before conception. Providing that her ultrasound examinations confirm normal growth without signs of either IUGR or macrosomia, and the fetal movement and CTG recordings remain normal I would defer delivery until 38 weeks. Although the onset of pulmonary maturity may be delayed in the fetus of a diabetic mother, at this gestation the risk of respiratory distress after delivery is small. Labour should be induced, caesarean section being indicated only if complications of labour demand operative intervention. In this case there are the other reasons discussed which make caesarean section particularly undesirable. The reason for advising induction of labour is the fear of antepartum stillbirth and the fact that this fetus has been exposed to a galaxy of medication including steroids, the effects of which on fetal well being are unpredictable. The diabetic control in labour would be achieved by the administration of an infusion of 10% glucose/insulin/potassium chloride mixture, the rate of infusion being determined by hourly BM stix estimation of the blood sugar together with confirmatory laboratory blood sugar estimations. Immediately after delivery of the placenta the insulin dosage is halved and the situation again monitored by regular estimation of the blood sugar until the oral intake is resumed and the twice daily administration of insulin recommenced.

Because of the antenatal administration of steroids hydrocortisone cover for labour will be required.

However well controlled the diabetes, the fetus is at risk for asphyxia and disproportion. Continuous fetal heart rate monitoring and resort to fetal scalp sampling when indicated are mandatory.

Discussion

Diabetes is associated with a threefold risk of congenital abnormality. The principal causes are neural tube defect (especially anencephaly), cardiac lesions, caudal regression and vertebral anomalies. The incidence of congenital abnormalities can be reduced by tight control of the diabetes immediately before and during the early weeks of pregnancy. Consequently elevated levels of HbA1 in the first trimester are correlated with an increased level of congenital malformations. After this, scrupulous control of the diabetes is designed to prevent fetal hyperglycaemia and hyperinsulinaemia with the sequelae of macrosomia, neonatal hypoglycaemia, polycythaemia, organomegaly and hyaline membrane disease from the disruption of surfactant metabolism. It also reduces the contribution to the perinatal mortality of the sudden and unexpected intrauterine death . Fetal hypoxia may be responsible in some cases, the maternal red cell oxygen transport is impaired when there are raised concentrations of glycosylated haemoglobin. Animal experiments suggest that fetal hyperglycaemia results in a lactic acid acidosis that can be sufficient to kill the fetus. Fetal hyperinsulinism may produce fetal hypoglycaemia if the delivery of glucose from the mother is rapidly reduced, e.g. during a hypoglycaemic attack. In this case reduced maternal insulin requirement and hypoglycaemia was taken as sufficient reason to deliver the baby.

The case presented concerns the management of a known insulin-dependent (established) diabetic. Pregnancy is diabetogenic and may precipitate diabetes for the first time during pregnancy. This may persist after delivery or resolve completely although these patient are likely to develop frank diabetes at a later date. Gestational diabetes therefore should be considered as glucose intolerance appearing during pregnancy. In strict and pedantic terms the gestational diabetic reverts to normal after pregnancy but this is a useless restriction demanding a retrospective diagnosis. Diabetes arising in pregnancy may be symptomatic with thirst, weight loss, polyuria and usually glycosuria but it can be asymptomatic. Whichever presents both are associated with an increased perinatal mortality. If a symptomatic patient has a random venous plasma glucose level of $\geqslant$11.0 mmol/l then she has diabetes mellitus. A fasting sample with a level of 8.0 mmol/l or above is equally diagnostic. Random levels $<$8.0 or fasting levels $<$6.0 mmol/l exclude the condition.

The problem lies in establishing glucose intolerance in the asymptomatic patient during pregnancy. This usually involves subjecting the patient to some form of glucose challenge and unfortunately the literature abounds with conflicting advice as to which test should be used. It is reasonable to quote the recommendations of the WHO Expert Committee on Diabetes Mellitus (1980) even though they were not addressing themselves to the state of pregnancy alone. If a fasting plasma glucose concentration is $>$8.0 mmol/l and/or the 2-h concentration following a 75 g oral glucose load is $>$11.0 mmol/l then diabetes is diagnosed. This definition creates a middle ground where the fasting level is $<$8.0 mmol/l but the 2-h result lies between 8.0 mmol/l and 10.9 mmol/l, such cases are diagnosed as 'impaired glucose tolerance'.

The benefit of the tight control of established diabetes is accepted. The value of treating the asymptomatic gestational diabetic in terms of reducing the perinatal mortality is less obvious although it probably reduces the incidence of macrosomia. Treatment ranges from the modification of the diet to the use of insulin or both.

Nevertheless, there is a body of opinion to screen the obstetric population to detect asymptomatic gestational diabetes. At its simplest this consists of subjecting women with specific features in their past history or certain physical characteristics to random blood sugar testing in pregnancy. This is usually carried out at booking. The criteria include a history of stillbirth, neonatal death or recurrent fetal loss at any gestation, past fetal abnormality, previous inappropriate fetal weight for gestation or size of patient, unexpected neonatal RDS, past gestational diabetes, a booking weight in excess of 90 kg or inappropriate weight for height, a maternal family history of diabetes or a history of glycosuria. For such patients, the test would be repeated at 32–34 weeks. Other patients would be recruited in the event of hydramnios, suspected macrosomia, suspected fetal abnormality or glycosuria. Testing should be repeated later in pregnancy in any patient where the suspicion of gestational diabetes persists, because the condition can develop late in pregnancy. A result of more than two standard deviations of the unselected clinic population indicate a formal oral glucose tolerance test.

Glycosuria will develop in 50% of all pregnant women at some time, and not all women with gestational diabetes will develop glycosuria. Similarly 10% of a normal Caucasian population will have babies weighing 4.5 kg or more.

Because of this imprecision, screening of the whole antenatal population has been advocated by others. Some advise random blood sugar estimations at booking and between 28 and 32 weeks, values above two standard deviations for the population again demanding referral for a full oral glucose tolerance test. Because there is much difference of opinion as to what constitutes a 'meal' and the patients are often uncertain of its timing others suggest that each patient should receive an oral glucose load on their arrival for the first time at the clinic and have a random blood sugar taken 1 h later. If this value exceeds the limits for the population then an OGTT is performed. If the test is normal the screening test is repeated at 28 weeks gestation as it is in those patients with criteria of increased risk for gestational diabetes. Positive screening tests are again followed by an OGTT. Using such criteria, between 1% and 2% of a clinic population have been found to have unsuspected diabetes at booking or developing during pregnancy. There is a danger that by setting a final 'screening' test at an arbitrary date of 28 weeks, a negative result implies that the possibility of gestational diabetes can be safely disregarded. This is unwise as the condition can develop late and further screening should take place if the clinical picture is at all suggestive.

Each of these alternatives have their own vigorous proponents but more often than not the management selected depends upon such pragmatic limitations as the clinic size, the number of personnel and financial limits.

Comment

This was a complicated history to take and deliver. The examiners would take this into account and the quality of the history would particularly influence their mark. The candidate should search out such information that would dictate management, e.g. changes in the insulin requirement even though this may well not be volunteered by the patient.

The topic of gestational diabetes is controversial. The candidate must be aware of the principles involved and have some opinion on the options he would adopt given free choice. He should be thoroughly familiar with the system used in his own hospital.

Outcome

The decision of the team in charge of the case was to await the spontaneous onset of labour. At 37 weeks the patient's insulin requirement inexplicably began to fall and she experienced one or two episodes of hypoglycaemia. Preprandial blood sugars of 4.5, 6.5 and 3 mmol/l and a fasting blood sugar of 2.3 mmol/l were obtained on an insulin dosage at 07.30 hours: Actrapid 6 units/Monotard 20 units; 17.30 hours: Actrapid 20 units only. This change was interpreted as reflecting some change in the fetomaternal balance and labour was induced. The blood sugar level at induction of labour was 4.5 mmol/l. An infusion of 8 units of Actrapid insulin and 20 mmol of KCl in 500 ml of 10% dextrose was administered by infusion pump at a rate of 1 unit per hour. This resulted in hourly blood sugar levels of between 8 mmol/l and 9 mmol/l throughout labour. Hydrocortisone 50 mgm i.v. was given at induction of labour and 25 mgm i.v. given every 6 h thereafter until oral therapy was possible. Attempts to site an epidural anaesthetic were unsuccessful. After rupture of the membranes labour supervened rapidly. No augmentation was required and after a first stage of 2 h she was delivered of a female infant weighing 3120 g with an Apgar score of 9 at 1 min. The baby required no further medical attention. The patient experienced an 800 ml postpartum haemorrhage which was controlled by giving ergometrine 0.5 mg i.v.

Further reading

BEARD, R. W., GILLMER, M. D. G., OAKLEY, N. W. and GUNN, P. J. (1980) Screening for gestational diabetes. *Diabetes Care*, **3**, 468–471

DRURY, M. I. (1986) Management of the pregnant diabetic – are the pundits right? *Diabetologia*, **29**, 10–12

LIND, T. and McDOUGALL, A. N. (1981) Antenatal screening for diabetes mellitus by random blood glucose sampling. *British Journal of Obstetrics and Gynaecology*, **88**, 346–351

LOWY, C. and BEARD, R. W. (1982) Report to the meeting on the results of the UK survey of diabetic pregnancies. Royal College of Obstetricians and Gynaecologists, London

Case 26

The 25-year-old housewife was seen routinely in the gynaecological clinic having been referred by her GP with a history of vaginal discharge and premenstrual headache. She had discontinued the oral contraceptive 6 months earlier because of the fear of possible complications. The couple were using sheaths for contraception. Her periods had become heavier but had remained regular, 6/30. Her headache was symmetrical across the forehead but sometimes extended over the crown as well. There was no nausea or vomiting but at its worst strong light aggravated the situation. There were no other visual disturbances. The headache constantly developed on days 21 or 22 of the cycle, gradual at first but becoming maximal a week later. The subsequent 48 h until the onset of the period was particularly bad and she had learnt to limit her activities at this time. Her symptom was relieved with the onset of the period. The intensity of the symptoms varied from cycle to cycle but some headache was invariable. She also complained of abdominal distention which commenced the week before the onset of the period and for the week after its completion. It could also develop at other times in the cycle and for varying lengths of time. Since stopping the oral contraceptive the periods had become more painful. Lower abdominal pain started 24–48 h before the onset of bleeding. It was cramp-like in nature and remained localized to the hypogastrium. The pain resolved almost completely by the end of the first day.

Her vaginal discharge was described as yellowish and sufficient to stain her underclothing. There had never been any blood in the discharge. The loss was not offensive or irritative. The GP had treated this with clotrimazole but to no effect. A cervical smear had been taken and reported as showing mild dyskaryosis suggestive of CIN I.

The menarche had been at 13 years of age and she felt that initially her periods had been unremarkable. She married at 17 years of age and fell pregnant quickly having a baby the following year. The pregnancy was normal as was the delivery. She took the combined oral contraceptive without concern until electively stopping it to conceive again. This baby was delivered after a normal pregnancy and confinement 18 months ago. She recommenced the same oral contraceptive preparation until stopping it as described. Systematic enquiry failed to elicit any further symptomatology.

Her past history was uncomplicated apart from an admission shortly after the most recent confinement for an overdose following marital and in-law problems. She was on no medication.

On examination she was normotensive, BP 120/65 mmHg. Her general examination was satisfactory. A neurological examination confirmed normal and symmetrical reflexes. There were no localizing signs on examining the cranial nerves and the optic fundi were grade 0. On palpation of the abdomen there was a soft poorly defined mass the size of an orange in the right iliac fossa. It was slightly tender and fixed. The genitalia were normal apart from the scar of a previous episiotomy. On speculum examination a healthy-looking cervix was visualized with an extensive ectopy. There was copious clear mucus. On bimanual examination the uterus was of normal size anteverted and mobile. A mass approximately 11 cm in diameter was palpable above, someway behind, separate from, and to the right of the uterus. The uterus could be moved independently of the mass which was relatively fixed.

Questions

From the history and the examination what lines of enquiry do you wish to pursue?

It is difficult to unite the problems presented into a single diagnosis. The symptoms of which the patient complains, i.e. headache and vaginal discharge are probably unrelated to the two features which would preoccupy the gynaecologist, namely the abdomino/pelvic mass and the abnormal cervical smear.

The nature of the mass is uncertain. Its position is rather high for an ovarian lesion but does not exclude it. The patient reports very few symptoms but does complain of abdominal distention not specifically related to the menses. There is no history of change in bowel habit or darkened stool but a caecal tumour, regional ileitis, or old appendix abscess might account for the mass. Another alternative might be a pelvic kidney. An abdomino/pelvic ultrasound would be of assistance in the first instance. An absent kidney on the right side at its normal location would strongly suggest a pelvic kidney, although it is possible for a pelvic kidney to coexist with another kidney on the same side. The normal ovary might be identified separately or an ovarian cyst demonstrated. If the ultrasound is equivocal then an IVU and barium enema should exclude or confirm the diagnosis. The signs are not suggestive of chronic pelvic inflammatory disease with pyo/hydrosalpinx. Neither are they consistent with a fibroid nor a paraovarian cyst. The patient complains of discharge but she has never been constitutionally unwell and the discharge of which she complains has never caused irritation or been offensive in odour. A full blood count and ESR would be helpful. If the issue then remains uncertain a laparotomy would be appropriate.

Why not laparoscopy?

Apart from a pelvic kidney all the other lesions listed for the differential diagnosis represent significant pathology. An IVU would certainly identify a functioning pelvic kidney; if non-functional then it ought to be removed. If the mass is tubal or ovarian then surgical treatment is required and laparoscopy merely delays the management. If the problem lies in the bowel then laparoscopy has little to offer from the point of view of diagnosis. With an uncertain diagnosis laparotomy should be arranged with the necessary surgical or urological expertise available.

What about the abnormal cervical smear?

The cervix looks healthy with no obvious signs of infection. At examination I would have taken the appropriate swabs to identify the gonococcus, *Chlamydia, Trichomonas, Gardnerella, Candida* and bacterial infection. These will likely be reported negative. On the combined pill cervical secretions are reduced because of the continuous influence of progesterone. When the patient reverted to her normal cycle, and with a significant degree of ectopy, it is not surprising that in mid cycle she became aware of a surge in her natural cervical secretions under the influence of oestrogen. If the bacteriological examinations were reported positive then I would treat the specific infection and repeat the smear. If the screen were reported negative I would undertake colposcopy and microbiopsy.

The smear shows only the lowest grade of dyskaryosis, why not wait a while and repeat it?

It is true that in a significant number of patients with this degree of abnormality the cervical smear will revert to normal over time, although the exact proportion of those that regress varies considerably in different reports. Colposcopy is not a pleasant experience and generates its own spectrum of anxiety and psychosexual trauma in some patients. There is an argument therefore simply to keep these patients with mildly dyskaryotic smears under cytological revue and to refer for colposcopy only those cases where the abnormality persists. However, a cervical smear can show mild dyskaryosis when a colposcopic biopsy identifies CIN III or even an invasive lesion. The usual criterion for the diagnosis of disease regression is the finding of two consecutive negative smears after the abnormal presenting smear. In prospective studies combining colposcopy with cytology, cytological regression has been diagnosed despite the persistence of colposcopic abnormality. There are also conflicting reports about the rate of progression of some of these milder atypia. It has been suggested that in some young women the transit time from CIN I to CIN III may be much more rapid than was previously appreciated. There has also been a threefold rise in the cervical cancer mortality for young women under 35 years of age. Because of these uncertainties I would advise that this patient be referred for definitive diagnosis by histology of a colposcopic biopsy.

What about the patient's presenting symptoms?

The question of the vaginal discharge has been partially dealt with. If there is infection then specific treatment should be prescribed. If the colposcopic examination proves to be completely clear then she can be reassured that her discharge is physiological and reflects a return to her natural hormonal milieu following the cessation of the oral contraceptive. If nevertheless she still seeks symptomatic relief then cryotherapy to the ectopy should solve the problem. In the event of dysplasia being detected in the cervix then ablation of the transformation zone would solve the problem with leucorrhoea also.

Her other symptoms are more problematical. The 'bloatedness' is not related to her menses and occurs at all times in the cycle. The headaches, however, are migrainous in nature and appear to be genuinely associated with the approach and onset of the menses resolving soon after their onset. She also has a degree of dysmenorrhoea. The pattern of her migrainous attacks and their onset with the cessation of ovulatory suppression is consistent with true premenstrual syndrome. It is true that she has had to cope with many stresses and that she was admitted with an overdose in the puerperium. The details of this admission are not available but it is known that puerperal depression is commoner in women who subsequently develop PMS. It is unusual that her symptoms are restricted almost completely to headache without any other associated symptoms. There are behavioral changes in that she takes to her bed, stays at home and limits her activities but this seems to be directly related to the severity of the headache.

How would you treat this patient?

In view of the severity of the headache and the limitations of a gynaecologist's neurological examination I think that it would be advisable to solicit the opinion of a neurologist. If no underlying neurological cause is defined then it is the evaluation of the pelvic mass and cervical dysplasia that take precedent. Symptomatic relief could be obtained by prescribing once more the oral contraceptive to inhibit ovulation until such diagnoses have been established and dealt with. If the symptoms persist after ovulatory suppression then the underlying problem is not PMS. If the patient prefers alternative treatment at that stage then the management is more difficult. There are many theories as to the aetiology of PMS but none explain all of the variations that present. There is therefore a spectrum of treatments available, few of which have been subjected to clinical trials, and which are therefore empirical. It is often a matter of ringing the changes to find which preparation gives the patient the best relief. Alternate treatments include the prescription of diuretics, bromocriptine, pyridoxine. mefenamic acid and dydrogesterone all of which have been shown to have advantages over placebo for some of the symptoms that these sufferers exhibit. The claims are difficult to interpret because placebo itself will cause some symptomatic relief in half the patients.

Discussion

There is a great deal of discussion currently about the proper management of the mildly abnormal cervical smear suggesting CIN I. Unfortunately this is resulting in some polarization of attitudes represented by cytopathologists on the one hand and gynaecologists on the other. The concerns of the gynaecologist were expressed by the candidate. There is no doubt that to refer all cases with mild dyskaryosis for colposcopy would in some areas stretch the colposcopy service to breaking point and therefore there is some pressure to avoid this. The alternative recommended is to repeat the cervical smear 3 months later and to refer the patient for colposcopy if abnormalities persist. There can be no doubt that the major contribution to any reduction in the incidence and mortality from cervical cancer has been through the adoption of population cervical screening. But colposcopy is not in competition with cytology in this respect. The initial key to management is and will continue to be the reading of an abnormal cervical smear. Colposcopy is purely a technique to provide the histological diagnosis while avoiding the morbidity of cone biopsy. It is true that colposcopic biopsies are sometimes difficult to read and provide their own problems with false positive and false negative results but this is no more than for cytological diagnosis in the first instance. Colposcopy is an invasive and unpleasant experience for most patients and generates its own legacy of anxiety and even psychosexual damage. Much is made of this by those who advocate purely cytological follow up of mildly abnormal smears. However, repeating a smear is not without its own problems from this point of view, particularly when it has been the vogue to refer to the taking of a 'cancer' smear. There are even now significant numbers of women who evade screening programmes and default from cytological follow up not only in hospitals but well women clinics, family planning clinics and GPs surgeries. It is somewhat arrogant to suppose that gynaecologists working in the field do not sympathise with and are not aware of the implications of their management. The answer lies not in the techniques applied but in comprehensive health education and an informed clientele as well as a sensitivity to the patient's concerns by those delivering the service. The question to be asked is whether that degree of disruption occasioned by colposcopy is justified to identify the very few women with a mildly abnormal smear who harbour a CIN III lesion, or even more rarely an invasive lesion. The efficacy of surveillance by cytology depends upon the patient's compliance in attending for follow-up. This varies enormously depending on many factors including the socioeconomic status of the patients. Generalities about management can therefore be misleading and units will be best advised to audit their own situation and decide about the management of these patients after considering the facilities available for colposcopy, the compliance of the patients and the performance of the cytological laboratory in terms of quality assessment. If, when comprehensive cervical screening is achieved, there is the corresponding reduction in incidence and mortality from cervical cancer hoped for, then the few cases that will develop cervical cancer while under cytological review will become unacceptable. Perhaps the best alternative is to apply the optimal management with colposcopic examination from the outset. In the meantime in view of the conflicting data available there is a good case to address the problem by establishing a multicentre prospective study for the management of patients presenting with mildly abnormal cervical smears.

The questions of clinic load and patient compliance are also responsible for two modes of patient management in colposcopy clinics. The usual approach is to perform colposcopy and microbiopsy and then recall the patient for ablative therapy when the biopsy results and the repeat cytology report is available. The concern is that without this sequence invasive lesions may be treated unknowingly or that treatment may be applied unnecessarily. The opposite argument for treatment at the time of biopsy is that once the biopsy result is available the treatment can be augmented later if necessary and that there is no danger of a patient not receiving treatment who requires it. Should the patient then default treatment has been given. Furthermore, treatment at the time of biopsy reduces the number of attendances at the clinic and increases the throughput. A compromise is to have a senior histopathologist in attendance at colposcopy clinics to report on frozen section biopsy material so that cervical ablation can be applied after microbiopsy. This is a luxury that few centres can realise and represents an enormous waste of consultant resources when other options are available.

This debate has to some extent been resolved by the emergence of a technique which both achieves a definitive biopsy and treats the lesion at one and the same time. This is the technique of Large Loop Excision of the Transformation Zone (LLETZ). The accuracy of the traditional colposcopically-directed microbiopsy in diagnosing cervical abnormalities has depended upon the experience of the colposcopist and the adequacy of the biopsy. When the microbiopsy and the cytology are in accordance then the biopsy is usually considered to be adequate. Should the cytology reveal changes much more severe than the histology of the microbiopsy then either repeat examination or cone biopsy become necessary. With LLETZ the whole transformation zone (the area at risk) is removed and the specimen is available for histological examination. Sampling error is therefore reduced and incomplete removal of carcinoma *in situ* can be recognized. The technique provides comparable success rates for single treatment to other modalities for cervical ablation: radical diathermy, cryotherapy, laser or cold coagulation. In most cases therefore biopsy and treatment are achieved at the same visit. The clear advantage is that the removal of the transformation zone *in toto* alleviates the concern with microbiopsy that a more severe focus or even microinvasion may have been missed. This management safely satisfies the constraints imposed by clinic loads and any lack of patient cooperation for follow-up.

Comment

The candidate here is presented with the combination of a simple history and physical signs that do not fit. As a general rule multiple diagnoses are to be avoided but in this case there is no alternative. What is important is how the candidate responds, especially how he establishes his priorities for management.

Outcome

An ultrasound examination confirmed the absence of the right kidney at its usual location. A mass was identified separate from the ovary at the pelvic brim over the right sacroiliac joint. An IVU confirmed a functioning pelvic kidney. The renal tract on the left was normal. The patient was reassured that this need cause her no concern but that any urinary symptoms should be reported to her doctor immediately. The neurologist was unable to define any neurological defect but requested an EEG and skull CT scan. These were reported as normal. She was then placed on the combined oral contraceptive and her menstrual migraine resolved, although bloatedness remained a problem. Colposcopic biopsies confirmed the presence of CIN III in the cervix. The transformation zone was treated with CO_2 laser to a depth of

10 mm. Follow-up for 2 years was negative. She then discontinued the oral contraceptive to achieve another pregnancy. She did not develop again the symptoms of PMS. She fell pregnant and aborted at 18 weeks. Further investigations confirmed a bicornuate uterus. She fell pregnant again and carried the baby to term.

Further reading

CAMPION, M. J., McCANCE, D. J., CUZIK, J. and SINGER, A. (1986) Progressive potential of mild cervical atypia: prospective cytological, colposcopic, and virological study. *Lancet*, **ii**, 237–240

PRENDERVILLE, W., CULLIMORE, J. and NORMAN, S. (1989) Large loop excision of the transformation zone (LLETZ). A new method of management for women with cervical intraepithelial neoplasia. *British Journal of Obstetrics and Gynaecology*, **96**, 1054–1060

ROBERTSON, J. H., WOODEND, B. E., CROZIER, E. H. and HUTCHINSON, J. (1988) Risk of cervical cancer associated with mild dyskaryosis. *British Medical Journal*, **297**, 2, 18–21

Case 27

The 28-year-old dental receptionist presented in her second pregnancy at 8 weeks by dates. Her cycle had been regular, 5/28, according to a carefully kept menstrual calendar.

Eight years ago after an uneventful pregnancy she went into spontaneous labour at 38 weeks gestation and was delivered normally of a boy weighing 3070 g. The puerperium was uneventful.

Four years later she developed a severe illness involving generalized arthralgia, escalating hypertension and renal dysfunction. A renal biopsy was performed and it revealed changes pathognomonic of systemic lupus erythematosus. The situation was controlled by a combination of immunosuppressive and antihypertensive therapy. When the disease had been in remission for 2 years the couple sought advice as to the wisdom of further pregnancies. After counselling they decided to embark on the current pregnancy. Her blood pressure had been controlled by an ACE inhibitor (angiotensin converting enzyme inhibitor) but before conception this was changed to methyldopa. She took a maintenance dose of prednisolone 5 mg daily.

At the booking visit her general examination was satisfactory and the pelvic examination confirmed an intrauterine pregnancy of a size consistent with her dates. At that time her blood pressure was 130/85 mmHg. Her dose of methyldopa was 250 mg three times daily. She was booked for hospital antenatal care and seen fortnightly to 24 weeks and weekly thereafter. At 15 weeks for 7 days she experienced intermittent vaginal bleeding which resolved spontaneously after resting in bed on the advice of her GP. An ultrasound examination at 18 weeks confirmed an apparently normal singleton fetus of a size appropriate to dates. Ultrasound examinations were repeated at monthly intervals and cardiotocography weekly from 30 weeks. The pregnancy appeared to progress normally to 33 weeks when auscultation of the fetal heart detected a bradycardia of 60 beats/min. Cardiotocography revealed that the fetal bradycardia was episodic lasting up to 10 min at a time. The episodes were unrelated to uterine activity. She had felt entirely well and there had been no further vaginal bleeding. An ultrasound examination on admission confirmed consistent growth with no suggestion of IUGR or asymmetry.

She is now at 34 weeks gestation. Her BP is 150/105 mmHg. The uterine size is consistent with dates. There is a single fetus and the lie is longitudinal. The head is not engaged in the pelvis. The back is on the left and the fetal heart is auscultated at a rate of 124 beats/min and regular. There is no peripheral oedema. The optic fundi are normal. Her tendon reflexes are normal and symmetrical. The urine contains protein + on testing with the dipstick provided. There is no haematuria.

Questions

Summarise this case from the history you have obtained.

This patient is in her second pregnancy at 34 weeks gestation. She is known to have had systemic lupus erythematosus with renal impairment. She has been admitted with a history of fetal heart irregularity. Her BP is significantly raised.

Was the decision advising this woman to become pregnant a wise one?

The prognosis for SLE in pregnancy is uncertain. The disease can exacerbate especially in the puerperium. The majority of pregnancies succeed when, as in this case, the disease has been quiescent for at least 6 months before conception. This applies even if there were severe changes in the original renal biopsy and proteinuria were heavy in the early stages of the disease. If there were evidence of persistent active disease or renal disfunction at booking, then a complicated pregnancy with deterioration in the maternal condition and a high risk of fetal loss would be probable and a therapeutic abortion might be offered.

These are the results of some tests obtained at booking and at the time of her admission at 33 weeks. What was the renal status at booking? What results were reassuring?

	At booking	33 Weeks
Routine haematology:	Normal	Normal
24-h creatinine clearance:	105 ml/min	55 ml/min
24-h urinary protein:	0.6 g	0.7 g
Plasma creatinine:	80 μmol/l	150 μmol/l
Plasma urea:	4.9 mmol/l	9.6 mmol/l
VDRL test:	Positive	Positive
Fluorescent *treponema* antibody absorption test (FTA – abs):	Negative	Negative
Anticardiolipin antibody (N = < 50)	75	80
Anti-Ro(SS-A) antibody:	Present	Present
Lupus anticoagulant (APTT > 40 s):	Absent	Absent

At booking her blood pressure was satisfactory, albeit controlled with methyldopa in low dosage and certainly safe for pregnancy. Her renal function was satisfactory but the plasma creatinine of 80 μmol/l was above the normal range for early pregnancy (45–70 μmol/l). Nevertheless, the level was less than 125 μmol/l so that any renal dysfunction could only be classified as mild. The proteinuria was insignificant.

What change had occurred in the renal status by 33 weeks?

The 24-h creatinine clearance has been halved, a drop of greater magnitude and earlier than the normal 15–20% fall experienced in the last few weeks of a normal pregnancy. It represents severe renal deterioration and this is reflected in plasma creatinine (150 μmol/l) and plasma urea (9.6 mmol/l). Her proteinuria however has remained virtually unchanged. There is now significant hypertension. Without the history the combination of hypertension and renal dysfunction might be mistaken for pre-eclampsia rather than a relapse of her SLE nephropathy.

What are your options for management?

It might be possible to modify the renal deterioration by a much increased dosage of steroids. Likewise the blood pressure might be controlled by increasing the amount of methyldopa or employing some other hypotensive. At this gestation further control of the hypertension is unlikely to improve the fetal prognosis significantly and in the presence of deteriorating renal function is inadvisable. There also remains the problem with the fetal heart rate which is atypical in that the episodes of bradycardia are prolonged and not related to uterine activity. The time has come to deliver the baby.

Do any of the results given offer an explanation for the fetal heart pattern?

Congenital heart block is usually found in association with either structural congenital heart abnormalities or connective tissue disease in the mother. In the CTD disorders the block may be partial, complete, or episodic. In SLE a wide spectrum of antibodies may be detected in the maternal serum. IgG crosses the placenta and it is postulated that the antibodies initiate the formation of immune complexes which locate on the cardiac conducting system disrupting normal function. In SLE anti-Ro (SS-A) antibody (antibody to soluble ribonuclear protein) is almost always present when there is heart block in the neonate. This antibody is found in approximately a quarter of patients with the disease.

How would you evaluate the fetal heart further?

Echocardiography and detailed ultrasound of the fetal heart should at this gestation identify major structural abnormalities; and by measuring the atrial and ventricular rates, any dissociation between the two confirming a conduction defect.

Was the bleeding in the second trimester of any special significance?

Possibly, rates of 40% have been quoted for pregnancy loss by abortion in women with SLE. The abortion tends to occur later than usual between the 12th and the 28th week of gestation. Recurrent pregnancy loss of this kind is an indication to seek serological evidence of the disorder. This phenomenon may present before the mother develops the overt disease.

Assuming that a degree of congenital heart block has been confirmed, how would you undertake delivery and do you anticipate any difficulties in management?

The patient has had a previous uneventful delivery. The presentation of the fetus is cephalic. Induction of labour with a view to a vaginal delivery is appropriate. Labour should be covered by parenteral hydrocortisone 100 mg i.m. 6-hourly. Although her hypertension is ascribed to renal disease rather than pre-eclampsia an epidural anaesthetic would be valuable to prevent escalation of the blood pressure with pain. This is assuming that her reported normal haematological values include a normal platelet count.

Under normal conditions where there is any concern for the fetus, fetal well-being in labour is assessed by continuous fetal heart monitoring and fetal scalp sampling when indicated. With a variable degree of heart block interpretation of the trace would be difficult and fetal assessment should be by elective serial fetal scalp samples at approximately 4-hourly intervals. Caesarean section would only be indicated on obstetric grounds. The puerperium is often the time when relapses of the underlying disease occur. This is when the majority of maternal deaths occur usually from pulmonary haemorrhage or pneumonitis. In this patient there has already been an exacerbation and the administration of high doses of steroids after delivery would seem a wise precaution.

Discussion

SLE is not uncommon. The incidence is approximately one in 700 women aged 15–64 years and is commoner in non-Caucasians. It is associated with a considerable fetal mortality, especially in the middle and last trimester. This loss is maximal when the disease is active but is also much increased when clinically the underlying condition is quiescent.

The disorder is characterized by the development of a spectrum of autoimmune antibodies the bulk of which are gamma immunoglobulins. These can cross the placenta and providing there is an expression of the appropriate antigen in the fetus produce an effect. From the point of view of pregnancy the following antibodies are of particular significance. These antibodies may be detected singly or together in individual cases.

Anti-Ro and anti-La (antibodies to soluble tissue ribonucleoprotein) are implicated in the pathogenesis of congenital heart block. Anti-Ro is found in 25% of the patients. After transplacental passage it initiates an immune inflammatory response in the fetal heart leading to fibrosis and calcification of the bundle of His, endocardioelastosis, cardiomyopathy and occasionally multiple structural abnormalities.

Cardiolipin is the antigen used for the VDRL screening test for syphilis. In the context of SLE, cardiolipin antibody refers to a positive test when syphilis has been excluded by the *Treponema pallidum* haemagglutination assay (TPHA) or fluorescent treponema antibody absorption test (FTA-abs). Detection of this antibody in early pregnancy has been associated with recurrent abortion, intrauterine death, pre-eclampsia, IUGR, and fetal distress. The higher the titre of anticardiolipin antibodies the greater the risk to the fetus.

Lupus anticoagulant (LE-anticoagulant) is something of a misnomer for the antibody detected in the serum of some women with the disorder. This acquired immunoglobulin is detected in about 9% of patients with SLE. It is an anti-phospholipid antibody which interferes with the activation of prothrombin by the prothrombin activator complex (factor Xa, factor V, calcium, and phospholipid). There is therefore prolongation of phospholipid-dependent coagulation tests such as the prothrombin time (PT), activated partial thromboplastin time (APTT), and kaolin cephalin clotting time (KCCT). Paradoxically, these patients do not show any tendency to a bleeding diathesis. The reverse is the case, a history of venous or arterial thrombosis is common. The complications of pregnancy listed for cardiolipin antibody apply also to LE-anticoagulant and high titres in pregnancy indicate a worsening prognosis for the fetus.

The mechanism by which these antibodies exert their effects is unclear. These anti-phospholipid antibodies do inhibit prostacyclin formation in vessel walls. This compound is a potent vasodilator and inhibitor of platelet aggregation. Thromboxane elaborated by platelets has precisely the opposite effect. Consequently, disruption of the prostacyclin/thromboxane balance would account for the thrombotic phenomena in the mother and the reduced platelet count observed in some cases. This mechanism has been postulated to explain the genesis of pre-eclampsia and IUGR both of which are commonly associated with fetal loss when the anti-phospholipid antibodies are present.

It is possible that anti-phospholipid antibody may account for some of the unexpected and unexplained fetal loss that occurs in pregnancy. Often a history of SLE has been obvious but sometimes the symptoms and signs may have been slight and not recognized.

Screening of maternal serum for cardiolipin antibody and LE-anticoagulant should be undertaken in pregnancy when there is a history of:

Unexpected second or third trimester fetal loss.
Recurrent first trimester abortion.
Deep vein or arterial thrombosis.
False positive VDRL test.
Reduced platelet count.
Clinical suspicion of SLE.

Which antibody is the best predictor of fetal outcome is uncertain. The evidence favours the IgG subtype of anti-cardiolipin, high titres indicating increased fetal risk, but differences in methodology make comparisons difficult.

It has been reported that treatment with aspirin and corticosteroids can improve the prognosis for the fetus when cardiolipin antibody or LE-anticoagulant is present in the maternal serum. The effect of treatment is monitored by the serial measurement of the KCCT. However, the patients may become Cushingoid at doses required to reduce the antibody titres and diabetes may be induced. Pre-eclampsia and/or IUGR may still develop and the closest fetal surveillance is required. Because of the side-effects of this therapy it has been suggested that those patients with a good obstetric history or who are nulliparous should receive aspirin only in the first instance, reserving steroids in addition for those patients with a bad obstetric history. A history of arterial or venous thromboembolism demands treatment with s.c. heparin for the duration of pregnancy.

The current mortality rate after delivery for infants with congenital heart block is 25%. There is no successful intrauterine therapy. Since the fetal cardiac conduction system is damaged the administration of medications to the mother in an attempt to increase the fetal heart rate will be unsuccessful. For those babies that survive there is often an improvement in cardiac performance after delivery and pacemakers are needed only in about 10–20%.

Intervention in the pregnancy is dictated by the severity of the maternal condition, especially the degree of hypertension or renal impairment as in this case or evidence of fetal compromise.

Comment

SLE is a condition that induces panic in candidates faced with a case in an examination. Possibly this is because the understanding of the disease is constantly evolving and demands some knowledge of autoimmune mechanisms. There is a tendency to categorize these problems as 'medical' and to consider it unfair to be presented with such a case in an obstetric examination. The obstetrician is however a doctor and it is unwise to close ones mind to developments in other fields especially where they impinge on obstetric practice. Even so the examiner starts by asking about the obstetric features of the case and providing data that is recognizable and pertinent. Only later, having satisfied himself that the candidate recognizes the obstetric implications of the case and has drawn the right conclusions from the information does he explore the medical dimension. Good answers here might lead to bonus marks.

Outcome

The patient was delivered by elective caesarean section of a female baby who weighed 2.18 kg. Despite the mother being on a long-term steroid regimen the baby developed severe RDS. The congenital heart block persisted and a pacemaker was introduced at 3 days of age after which the cardiac function stabilized.

Further reading

ESSCHER, E. and SCOTT, J. S. (1979) Congenital heart block and maternal systemic lupus erythematosus. *British Medical Journal,* **i**, 1235–1238

LOCKSHIN, M. D., DRUZIN, M. L., GOEI, S., QAMAR, T., MAGID, M. S., JOVANOVIC, L. and FERENC, M. (1985) Antibody to cardiolipin as a predictor of fetal distress or death in pregnant patients with systemic lupus erythematosus. *New England Journal of Medicine,* **313**, 152–156

LUBBE, W. F., BUTLER, W. S., PALMER, S. J. and LIGGINS, G. C. (1984) Lupus anticoagulant in pregnancy. *British Journal of Obstetrics and Gynaecology,* **91**, 357–363

Case 28

The 24-year-old shop assistant was admitted to the unit as an intrauterine transfer from her district hospital. It was her first pregnancy. She had originally booked late with a history of 21 weeks amenorrhoea. The uterine size at this time was considered to be more consistent with a 16-week pregnancy. An ultrasound scan confirmed this impression and her EDD was established a month later when a second scan demonstrated apparently normal incremental growth. The fetus appeared normal. At 28 weeks she was admitted to hospital with pregnancy-induced hypertension. Her BP was recorded as 135/100 mmHg, there was no proteinuria. She remained in hospital, her BP varying between 140/100 mmHg and 140/90 mmHg. She felt well throughout, her urine remained free of protein and her fluid output was sustained. At 31 weeks gestation she went into preterm labour. The diagnosis was established by progressive effacement and dilatation of the cervix as detected on vaginal examination. Dexamethasone was given and an attempt made to suppress uterine activity by the use of intravenous ritodrine. Despite the therapy she progressed to 4 cm dilatation and transfer was instituted. On arrival she was 6 cm dilated. The single fetus presented by the head. Her BP was 140/90 mmHg. It was decided to allow labour to proceed. The membranes were ruptured and clear liquor released; a clip electrode was applied to the fetal scalp for continuous fetal monitoring. Two hours later she had a spontaneous delivery of a male infant, weighing 1730 g, in good condition. The only analgesia she had required had been Entonox®. Her blood pressure had remained stable throughout labour and her fluid balance record was satisfactory. The first stage of labour had lasted 8 h and the second stage was completed in 35 min. An elective episiotomy was performed but otherwise no specific measures were taken to modify the delivery. The baby was transferred to the neonatal nursery. The mother's condition remained stable, her BP never rose above the admission value and she was transferred to the postnatal ward where, over 48 h, her blood pressure settled to booking values (120/70 mmHg). She elected to stay in the unit to remain near her baby who had now developed hyaline membrane disease.

Initially she remained completely fit but on day 6 felt generally unwell and particularly nauseous. Ward testing of the urine confirmed the presence of protein and on direct questioning she admitted to some dysuria. Her temperature was then recorded as 38.2°C. A sample of urine was sent for culture and antibiotic treatment commenced. Over the next 24 h she developed a headache mainly over the crown of the head but also at times occipital in its location. It has remained constant but not severe. In addition she finds bright lights uncomfortable. She is now 8 days postpartum. Her dysuria has resolved, her pyrexia persists, and the laboratory reports negative culture of the urine specimen.

On examination she is of normal habitus. Despite feeling nauseous she has continued to take fluid and there are no signs of dehydration. The tongue is moist and there is no skin laxity. Her face is 'puffy' and rather flushed, there is periorbital oedema. She is aware and communicative, although a little reluctant to move much with her headache. Speech is normal. There is no oedema of the hands, legs or sacrum. Her temperature is 38°C. Her BP is 120/65 mmHg and examination of the cardiovascular and respiratory systems is normal. Her extremities are normal there are no signs of deep vein thrombosis or thrombophlebitis. There is a small soft goitre with no bruit. She has an adhesive plaster on the right side of her neck. The breasts are normal and not engorged. She had elected not to breast feed, no anti-lactation drugs have been prescribed. The abdomen is slightly distended consistent with a recent pregnancy. There are striae gravidarum. The uterine fundus is just palpable at the symphysis pubis. It is not tender on palpation. There is no organomegaly and the renal angles are not tender. She is wearing a pad, the lochia, which is now slight, is not offensive. Inspection of the perineum shows that her episiotomy has healed well and cleanly;her sutures have been removed. Because of her headache she is reluctant to move her head but can put her chin on her chest. Kernig's sign is negative. The pupillary reflexes to light and accommodation are equal and symmetrical. There is some restriction to upward eye movement and to some extent lateral eye movement at the extremes of her range. She complains of no loss of visual acuity. There is no nystagmus. Examination of the optic discs is difficult because of her photophobia; there appears to be no papilloedema but the disc margins on both sides could be blurred medially. No signs of hypertensive retinopathy are seen. A systematic examination of cranial nerves V and VII – XII is normal. The ears and tympanic membranes appear healthy. Her tendon reflexes are equal and symmetrical. Her grip is slightly stronger on the right but she is right-handed.

Question

How would you summarize the situation you find?

This is a young primigravida who developed pregnancy-induced hypertension in early pregnancy. She went into preterm labour, was transferred to another hospital with neonatal facilities and delivered normally. The labour and delivery were uncomplicated. Her hypertension rapidly resolved. All was well until day 6 of the puerperium when she developed a postpartum pyrexia with symptoms initially of dysuria and nausea but later headache and photophobia. Her examination reveals nothing obvious to explain her pyrexia. A urinary tract infection has been excluded. Her history and examination suggest a cerebral complication but there are no localizing signs.

What do you mean by the term postpartum pyrexia?

The measurement of a temperature above 38°C following delivery.

In fact this is a technical term dating from the days when pelvic sepsis following delivery was a significant cause of maternal death. It was necessary to notify the Medical Officer of Health of any temperature reaching 100.4°F on any one occasion within 14 days of delivery. Under the rules of the then Central Midwives Board, midwives had to notify a doctor of any temperature of 99.4°F on three successive days during the lying-in period of 14 days and the Local Health Authority of any temperature of 100.4°F occurring within 21 days of childbirth or miscarriage. These rules were only rescinded in 1967.

How would you proceed with the management of this case?

The symptomatology does not lead to a specific diagnosis. She has a pyrexia and some of her symptoms could relate to infection. Her general malaise and nausea would fit into this category. On the other hand her periorbital oedema, suffusion of the face, photophobia, persistent headache and limited eye movements suggest cerebral pathology. I cannot at this stage suggest a single diagnosis to explain the total picture. The identification of a possible intracranial problem is the first priority. I would ask for the opinion of a neurologist immediately and request a skull X-ray and skull EMI scan to exclude an intracerebral lesion. Concurrently I would undertake a routine screen to identify possible infection.

How do you undertake such a screen?

I would start with a comprehensive physical examination as there may be more than one focus of infection. Because of the possible implications of puerperal infection for the future, bacteriological specimens should be submitted for examination even when there are no symptoms or signs attributable to a given system.

The immediate concern is to exclude genital tract infection. Swabs must initially be taken from the episiotomy site. It is then essential to pass a speculum to identify the cervix. Swabs for aerobic and anaerobic culture must be obtained from the cervix itself. Swabs for *Chlamydia* and *Neisseria gonorrhoeae* require special transport media. The commonest organisms include *E. coli, Proteus mirabilis, Bacteroides* spp., β-haemolytic streptococci and anaerobic streptococci (*Strep. faecalis*). It is the β-haemolytic streptococcus that most commonly colonizes the blood even when the primary site is not overtly established. All patients with a pyrexia above 39°C should have blood cultures taken. Less common organisms include *Neisseria gonorrhoeae, Pseudomonas aeruginosa and Clostridium perfringens.* If infection is suspected then empirical treatment with a combination of penicillin, 1 mega unit 6-hourly, and metronidazole 400 mg twice daily is appropriate. Except in a debilitated patient, extension of infection beyond the uterus rarely occurs before the second week and usually is prefaced by the signs of endometritis. The progression, is however, unpredictable and because the patient may deteriorate rapidly (especially with β-haemolytic streptococcal infection) empirical treatment is justified.

A carefully collected midstream specimen of urine should be collected into a sterile container. A sterile plug of gauze should be placed in the lower part of the vagina after vulval toilet and before the collection of the midstream specimen. The specimen is divided into two samples. The first is examined microscopically on the ward immediately after collection. The presence of pus cells indicates prompt antibiotic therapy pending the results of culture on the second sample. The commonest organisms are *E. coli, Strep. faecalis* and *Proteus.* Ampicillin or amoxycillin are useful first line antibiotics.

Attention should be directed to the breast. Breast infection usually occurs in the second postnatal week when the baby's pharynx has been colonized and the nipple traumatized by poor fixation of the baby to the breast. Samples of milk from an affected breast should be sent from culture and antibiotic sensitivity. A swab from the baby's pharynx should also be submitted. The organism is often a penicillin-resistant staphylococcus. First line treatment could be with ampicillin or flucloxacillin. Abscess formation demands surgical drainage.

If the patient had been delivered by caesarean section then a specimen of sputum should be sent for culture and if there are signs in the chest, a chest X-ray obtained. The wound must be inspected and swabs taken even if it means taking down a sealed dressing applied in theatre.

The examination should exclude non-infective causes of pyrexia such as deep vein thrombosis and superficial thrombophlebitis.

Would any blood tests assist you in the management of this case?

Probably not, a moderate leucocytosis and a raised ESR are usual after delivery. A very raised white cell count might suggest an infective focus. Electrolyte estimations would have been indicated had there been vomiting on any scale. Although not jaundiced, persistent nausea can be associated with liver dysfunction, and liver function tests would be helpful to exclude this possibility.

In fact the blood tests you describe were all negative as was a bacteriological screen for infection. An EMI scan and skull X-ray were performed as you suggested and were reported as normal. An EEG was reported as showing no focal abnormality. Why has this patient a dressing on her neck?

The patient did not volunteer any information and I did not specifically enquire as to the reason. In the context of the case possibly this was the site of carotid angiography.

The right carotid angiogram was reported as follows:

The appearances are consistent with superior sagittal sinus thrombosis, with blood clots in the transverse and sigmoid sinuses. There are prominent collateral channels draining blood downwards nearly all into the veins of the Sylvian fissure. No aneurysm or arteriovenous malformation has been shown. The internal cerebral vein and inferior sagittal sinus are more dilated than normal.

Can you tell me anything about sagittal sinus thrombosis and puerperal pyrexia?

No Sir.

Then let us explore something else.

Discussion

Primary cerebral venous thrombosis is a rare complication of pregnancy. It can be fatal and is sometimes associated with thrombosis at other sites. It is not to be confused with cerebral thrombophlebitis secondary to infections in the middle ear, face or skull. There is a probable association with pre-eclampsia. The most important guide to the diagnosis is an awareness of the condition and its special relationship to pregnancy and the puerperium. It should be suspected in any previously healthy woman who develops a syndrome of paresis, headache, vomiting, convulsions, speech difficulties and confusion after delivery. Thrombosis of the sagittal sinus is particularly associated with severe headache, nausea and vomiting, pyrexia and acute bilateral papilloedema. The face and scalp are often markedly congested and epistaxis is an occasional feature. Lumbar puncture may show a slight increase in CSF pressure but there are no specific changes in the fluid. It should be performed if meningitis cannot be excluded. An EEG, CT scan, or EMI investigation can be unhelpful. The diagnosis is established by carotid angiography. The treatment is not well established. Convulsions should be controlled using the usual agents. The case for anticoagulants is not clear cut. There is a fear that anticoagulation may in the acute phase lead to intracerebral haemorrhage or haemorrhagic infarction in relation to the venous thromboses. Low molecular weight dextran infusion may improve the cerebral blood flow. Mannitol infusion has been advocated to reduce cerebral oedema.

The puerperium is a phase of obstetric responsibility too often neglected by candidates and indeed doctors in general. Most complications that develop at this time are relatively minor and either resolve or are easily treated. Most candidates are completely ignorant as to the incidence of complications in the puerperium. With moves to delegate the discharge of postnatal patients to the midwifery staff there is an even greater temptation to consider the postnatal ward as being outside the province (and the responsibility) of the doctor. Failure to recognize infection in the early stages can have significant long-term sequelae especially in the genital tract where the result may ultimately be infertility. Most causes of pyrexia are easily attributable to the sequelae of childbirth or lactation but it is vital to consider unrelated causes of morbidity when the picture is obscure or atypical. Regular and frequent inspection of the postnatal patients helps to identify problems as they emerge and before they become serious.

Comment

This very unusual case was selected for presentation for two reasons. In the first instance it is not impossible for a postpartum patient to be presented in the examination. Second, although cerebral vein thrombosis is extremely rare and it is most unlikely that the candidate will ever have seen (or even perhaps heard of) such a case, the examiner is primarily interested in his approach to the problem. Candidates will not fail purely because they cannot diagnose the pathology. Particularly in the gynaecological cases the diagnosis may not have been established at the time of the examination and is equally unknown to the examiner.

Do not use complex terms where simple ones will do and avoid using terms with which one is not fully conversant. If the candidate had used the word 'temperature' rather than the phrase 'postpartum pyrexia' there would have been no idiosyncratic monologue on an item clearly close to the examiner's heart. This is important because it wastes time and leaves the candidate with less opportunity to display his knowledge.

The candidate here rightly declared the limits of his capability. Calling for another or more senior opinion is an established part of good practice. It might have been tempting to suggest a lumbar puncture in this case, a technique possibly within the compass of the candidate, but in such uncertain circumstances this would not have met with the examiner's approval. By avoiding this pitfall the candidates can direct the discussion to an area with which they are familiar.

When the diagnosis was revealed the candidate volunteered his complete ignorance of the condition. This is precisely the correct thing to do as long as this response does not recur too frequently in the viva! It is a most rare diagnosis and the examiner would not expect the candidate to be fully conversant with the condition. The examiner has two options, either to switch entirely to another topic related to the case or to coax some conjecture out of the candidate by referring to first principles with which he is familiar, e.g. the management of deep vein thrombosis in pregnancy.

By this time the candidate has established that he can investigate a difficult case in a logical, safe and rational manner. He certainly will not be penalized for lack of knowledge at this level.

An attempt to blunder on or to guess without further guidance from the examiner would create more problems than it would solve.

Outcome

For a short while the patient's symptoms increased, the headache becoming worse and papilloedema developing on the right side. Over 3 days the situation stabilized. The neurosurgical opinion was that as a good collateral circulation had established itself anticoagulants, streptokinase or thrombectomy were contraindicated. An ophthalmologist excluded any visual defect. Her symptoms gradually resolved over the next 7 days so that she was fit enough to return home. Six weeks later she was seen in the obstetric/medical clinic where she reported being entirely symptom free. Her examination was normal apart from some slight blurring of the disc margin on the right. An IUCD was fitted and she was advised not to pursue a pregnancy for at least 2 years and to contact the team before embarking on a pregnancy. It was explained that the oral contraceptive was not suitable for her. It was anticipated that repeat angiography before any decision about pregnancy would be advisable. Twelve weeks after this last visit she again developed headache and nausea this time with vomiting. Bilateral papilloedema was again present. She was started on anticoagulants and her symptoms again resolved. The baby continued to thrive.

Further reading

CARROLL, J. D., LEAK, D. and LEA, H. A. (1966) Cerebral thrombophlebitis in pregnancy and the puerperium. *Quarterly Journal of Medicine*, **139**, 347–367

Case 29

The patient had been seen first in the casualty department after an altercation with her boyfriend during which she was struck to the ground. Shortly afterwards she started to bleed per vaginum. The loss was painless and amounted to an 'egg cup full'. Her LMP had been 11 weeks before. On admission the casualty officer had taken blood for a routine haemoglobin estimation. The patient was seen by the gynaecological registrar who confirmed the clinical picture of a threatened abortion. An ultrasound examination identified an intrauterine pregnancy with a single active fetus with a CRL of 40 mm. The patient was reassured and as the bleeding had stopped allowed home.

The blood samples obtained in the casualty department were reported as follows:

Haemoglobin: 9.4 g/dl, Hct: 0.278, White blood cells: 12.7×10^9/l, Red blood cells: 2.58×10^{12}/l, MCV: 107.8 fl, MCH: 33.4 pg, MCHC: 33.8 g/dl, Platelets: 393×10^9/l, Reticulocytes: 11%, Film: Many reticulocytes and spherocytes. Multiple Howell Jolly bodies. The white cells are normal.

Because of these results the patient was admitted to hospital for further investigation.

The patient was 29 years of age and in her second pregnancy. Her first pregnancy 9 years before had been uneventful and at term she went into spontaneous labour and had a boy weighing 2807 g. The puerperium had been uneventful.

Since that pregnancy she had been entirely well and symptom free. Direct questioning excluded jaundice, anaemia, arthritis, ocular problems or skin changes. She took no drugs, did not smoke, and drank only a very occasional glass of wine. Her diet was normal and adequate. She had no known allergies. There was no relevant family history. This pregnancy was to a new partner. They had planned the pregnancy, an IUCD having been removed 2 months before her LMP. Her menstrual cycle had been regular.

On examination she was 158 cm in height and slight in build weighing 47.5 kg. Her conjunctiva were pale and the sclera clear. Her BP was 110/60 mmHg with a regular normal pulse of 80 beats/min. The mouth and tongue were normal, the thyroid was not enlarged. Her fingers and nails were unremarkable. Her abdomen was scaphoid, the uterine fundus was just palpable above the symphysis, the liver and spleen were not palpable. There were no petechiae or purpura. Examination of the CNS demonstrated no abnormalities. Pelvic examination confirmed an intrauterine pregnancy of a size consistent with her dates. A cervical smear was taken and this was reported as showing dyskaryosis suggestive of CIN II. She had not had a smear taken since her last pregnancy.

She was admitted to the ward. Further blood tests were performed and a marrow biopsy taken from the right iliac crest. After the results of the tests were assessed she received an infusion of freeze-dried immunoglobulin. A daily dose of 0.4 g/kg body weight was given as a 3% solution for 5 days. She was discharged home. Iron and folate supplements were prescribed.

She attended the antenatal clinic weekly thereafter. Ultrasound examination of the fetus was undertaken at 16, 23, 29 and 34 weeks.

At 16 weeks gestation prednisolone 30 mg daily was prescribed for her. This dose was reduced to 10 mg at 23 weeks, 5 mg at 24 weeks and discontinued a week later.

Colposcopic examination of the cervix was performed at 18 and 32 weeks gestation. She was told that an area of atypia was present and that it would be investigated further after delivery. No biopsies were taken.

Since 32 weeks she has been keeping a record of fetal movements on a kick chart. CTG recordings have been obtained at each antenatal visit and these have been reported as normal.

She is now at 36 weeks gestation, her general examination is as before except for the biopsy scar on the right hip. The uterine size is consistent with the gestational age. The fetus presents by the head which has not yet engaged in the pelvis. There is no excess liquor. The fetal heart is heard with a regular rate of 132 beats/min.

Questions

Clearly the findings on her routine blood analysis from the casualty department caused concern and she was admitted. What does the report indicate?

There is more than one abnormality. She is anaemic and at that gestation significant haemodilution would be unlikely. The reduced haematocrit would correlate with the reduced red cell count. The normal MCH and MCHC would exclude any significant degree of iron deficiency. The MCV is raised suggesting a megaloblastic normochromic anaemia but there is a marked reticulocytosis and no hypersegmented neutrophils have been reported in the blood film. Microspherocytes are usually a feature of red cell haemolysis.

What would be the first tests you would ask for?

Serum folate and B12 to exclude the commonest causes of megaloblastic anaemia. A direct Coombs test on the maternal erythrocytes would exclude autoimmune haemolytic anaemia and if there were any doubt still, a marrow biopsy would be indicated.

Here are some more results, what do they show?

Serum B12:	418 pg/ml (N = 160–600 pg/ml)
Serum folate:	9.8 ng/ml (N = 2.0–7.5 ng/ml)
Red cell folate:	744 ng/ml (N = 125–350 ng/ml)
Cardiolipin binding assay:	Negative
APTT:	Normal
Auto antibody screen [thyroid, (+ microsomes), ANA, reticulin, mitochondria, smooth muscle, gastric parietal cells, rheumatoid]:	Negative
Direct Coombs test:	IgG positive titre 1/32 IgA negative IgM negative C3d negative
LDH:	463 U/l (N = < 430 U/l)
Haptoglobin:	0.01 g/l (N = 1.0–3.0 g/l)
Serum albumin:	41 g/l (N = 34–50 g/l)
Serum alkaline phosphatase:	53 U/l (N = 30–130 U/l)
Serum total bilirubin:	20 µmol/l(N = < 17)
AST:	17 U/l (N = < 37)

Megaloblastic anaemia from folate or B12 deficiency is ruled out. The positive Coombs test is consistent with a haemolytic anaemia. The raised bilirubin suggests excess red cell destruction as does the raised LDH level. A normal serum AST level would exclude hepatocellular disease as a cause of the hyperbilirubinaemia. The antibody on the red cells is IgG. The antibody screen would exclude SLE as the cause of this autoimmune haemolytic anaemia. Autoimmune haemolytic anaemia in association with lupus usually involves both IgG and complement on the red cell. A reduced serum haptoglobin (haemoglobin binding protein) reflects the removal of the haptoglobin-haemoglobin complex by RE cells and the relatively low production of haptoglobin by the liver.

The megaloblastosis is still unexplained; an examination of the bone marrow might clarify the situation.

The marrow report showed increased cellularity. Erythropoiesis was prominent, myelopoiesis was normal. Megakaryocytes were healthy. Iron stores and sideroblasts were normal. The picture was entirely consistent with autoimmune haemolytic anaemia. Apart from B12 and folate deficiency what other causes of megaloblastic anaemia do you know?

Alcohol abuse, liver disease, myeloma, myelodysplastic disease, myxoedema, reticulocytosis, aplastic anaemia and cytotoxic drugs. None of these seems to apply in this case.

What are the implications for the fetus with autoimmune haemolytic anaemia in the mother?

I am not sure. The fetus will inherit red cell antigens from both mother and father. IgG is known to cross the placenta and consequently if the appropriate antigen is expressed in the fetus then antibody crossing from the mother might cause fetal red cell haemolysis in the same way as for Rhesus isoimmunization. This can certainly happen in mothers with autoimmune thrombocytopenia where placental transfer of antibody causes thrombocytopenia in the neonate.

How might you investigate the fetal situation?

Presumably the end result is fetal haemolysis and as in rhesus disease bilirubin will appear in the amniotic fluid. Amniocentesis and the spectrophotometric analysis of the amniotic fluid should identify any significant destruction of fetal blood. Amniocentesis however carries a small threat to the fetus. The relationship between antibody titre and the risk of fetal haemolysis has been well worked out for Rhesus disease and amniocentesis is often advised when the titre rises above 1/16. The significance of titres in this condition is not so established so that the timing of amniocentesis could be arbitrary. The degree of any haemolysis will increase with time. An amniocentesis now at 36 weeks will serve the dual purpose of estimating the degree of any effect and the fetal lung maturity – by L/S ratio measurement. The patient has had serial ultrasound examinations. The detection of fetal ascites or hydramnios by ultrasound earlier might have indicated amniocentesis or, as these signs would indicate severe changes, cordocentesis and possibly intrauterine transfusion.

So far her ultrasound examinations have remained satisfactory. Listed below are some more results. How do they relate to her history?

The patient received a course of i.v. gammaglobulin at 11 weeks gestation. She then received steroids between the 11th and the 16th weeks of gestation. Despite the giving of gammaglobulin at 11 weeks there was little change in the various indices. With the prescription of steroids however there was a rapid fall in the Coombs test titre. The haemoglobin level rose,although not dramatically, and the improvement in her anaemia was matched by a fall in the reticulocyte count. The MCV fell with the

Gestation (weeks)	*IgG titre*	*Hb* (g/dl)	*MCV* (fl)	*Platelets* ($\times 10^9$/l)	*Reticulocytes* (%)
12	1/32	9.3	107.2	409	12
14	1/32	9.2	104.4	388	13
16	1/32	10.2	106.4	375	12
18	1/16	10.5	100.8	347	4
20	1/4	11.0	94.9	388	2
22	1/2	10.7	93.9	367	2
26	1/1	10.6	90.6	255	1
30	1/1	10.1	91.7	312	2
34	1/32	9.9	93.0	330	3

improvement in the anaemia suggesting that this was a manifestation of the haemolytic change. The situation remained stable until 34 weeks when a rise in the direct Coombs IgG titre was accompanied by a rise in the reticulocyte count and the MCV suggesting an escape from the immunosuppression. The platelet counts show no particular trends.

This patient had an abnormal cervical smear in early pregnancy. How would you manage this problem?

The risk of this being associated with an invasive lesion is very small but nevertheless the possibility should be excluded. I would undertake a colposcopic examination at 16 weeks and repeat it at 3-monthly intervals. The cervix should be fully reassessed 3 months after delivery when involution is complete. At that visit colposcopic biopsies are taken of any atypical areas.

Would you take colposcopic biopsies?

Not routinely, the biopsies are small but the cervix is extremely vascular and troublesome haemorrhage may be encountered when the underlying disease is of minimal concern. Infection following biopsy is a further risk. I would rely on a careful colposcopic examination of the cervix. Usually pregnancy everts the cervical canal so that concerns about the visualization of the squamocolumnar junction are unlikely. If the appearances suggested that invasion were present or the colposcopic examination were inadequate by failure to delineate the whole lesion then a definitive biopsy would be essential either by cone or wedge biopsy. Because of the risk of haemorrhage such procedures should be conducted under general anaesthetic with an adequate supply of blood available for transfusion.

How and when would you deliver this baby?

The presence of cervical dysplasia does not contraindicate a vaginal delivery. She was seen first with a history of bleeding in early pregnancy and the effect of the maternal antibody on the fetus is unknown. I would plan to induce labour at 38 weeks to pre-empt any cumulative threat that these events might pose to the fetus. She will require steroid cover in labour. Hydrocortisone 100 mg i.m. 6-hourly for the duration of labour should be sufficient. Labour should be accompanied by comprehensive fetal monitoring. At delivery cord blood must be obtained for Coombs testing, haemoglobin and bilirubin estimations. Fresh blood compatible with the fetus should be available for transfusion or exchange transfusion if the indices suggest it. Unlike Rhesus isoimmunization the antibody is directed towards maternal non-blood group antigens. The effect of autoimmune antibodies on the fetal red cells is unpredictable, severe fetal haemolytic disease has been described but in many cases, despite high titres in the mother, the effect on the fetus is mild or may be absent.

Following delivery the maternal autoimmune haemolytic anaemia may persist or more commonly regress. Persistent disease would suggest ^{51}Chromium-labelled red cell survival studies to confirm haemolysis and to identify the sites of destruction, e.g. liver and/or spleen by surface counting.

Discussion

The usual treatment of autoimmune haemolytic anaemia is the giving of steroids. Patients with IgG only on the red cells usually respond better to steroids than those with IgG and/or complement or IgA. The diagnosis of autoimmune haemolytic anaemia was made in early pregnancy and in animal studies steroids have been associated with the induction of cleft palate abnormalities. Because of this concern about teratogenesis with the giving of steroids, an attempt was made to suppress the haemolytic process by giving i.v. immunoglobulin.

In the early 1980s reports appeared describing the effectiveness of i.v. monomeric polyvalent human immunoglobulin (IVIgG) in elevating the platelet count in immune thrombocytopenia. The mode of action is unclear. It has been demonstrated that the presence of high circulating antibody levels block the Fc receptors of the mononuclear – phagocyte system prolonging the survival of red cells carrying bound antibody. There may also be a degree of competitive inhibition with the autoimmune antibody at the target antigen. Autoimmune haemolytic anaemia responds less readily to IVIgG than does ITP.

If a colposcopic examination for an abnormal smear suggests that the basement membrane has been breached and invasion is present then a definitive biopsy is required. The patient's management then depends on the histological report. If the lesion is a microinvasive carcinoma with stromal invasion to a depth < 3 mm, and it has been removed *in toto*, then pregnancy might reasonably be allowed to proceed to term. Even so, if vascular or lymphatic channels contain tumour cells then a radical approach is necessary.

The management of an invasive lesion depends on the stage of the disease and the period of gestation at which the problem is diagnosed. For stage Ib and IIa disease the treatment should be surgical with the conservation of the ovaries in young women. In early pregnancy a radical Wertheim-type hysterectomy should be performed with the fetus *in situ*. If the gestation is such that the fetus is viable then the baby should first be delivered by caesarean section and then the surgeon proceeds to the radical procedure. In the presence of invasive disease there is no place for vaginal delivery. The risks include the dissemination of malignant cells from the cervix and catastrophic haemorrhage. For the more advanced stages of the disease the treatment is by radiotherapy. If the fetus is viable the radiotherapy follows classical caesarean section. If early, the treatment will induce an abortion after which an intracavitary source might be employed.

Outcome

Plans were made for this patient to undergo amniocentesis but before this could be performed she went into spontaneous labour at just 37 weeks gestation. After a short labour of five and a half hours she was delivered of a boy weighing 2650 g and with a cord blood pH of 7.44. The placenta weighed 500 g and appeared normal. The cord blood results were: Coombs test, positive; Hb, 12.6 g/dl; bilirubin, 41 μmol/l. The maximum recorded bilirubin level was 77 μmol/l 24 h after delivery. Transfusion was considered unnecessary.

Six days after delivery the maternal Hb was 9.6 g/dl, the MCV was 92 fl and the reticulocyte count 3%.

Further reading

CHAPLIN, H., COHEN, R., BLOOMBERG, G., KAPLAN, H. J., MOORE, J. A. and DORNER, I. (1973) Pregnancy and idiopathic autoimmune haemolytic anaemia: a prospective study during 6 months gestation and 3 months postpartum. *British Journal of Haematology*, **24**, 219–229

NEWLAND, A. C. (1989) The use and mechanisms of action of intravenous immunoglobulin: an update. *British Journal of Haematology*, **72**, 301–305

SHEPHERD, J. S. (1985) Cancer complicating pregnancy. In *Clinical Gynaecological Oncology* (eds J. S. Shepherd and J. M. Monaghan), Blackwell Scientific, Oxford, Ch. 16

Case 30

The 82-year-old lady was well known in her village community for her many activities, not the least riding her bicycle from one meeting to another. She lived alone but close by was her married daughter. She was referred to the hospital by her GP. Her principal complaint was incontinence of urine. Despite her sprightliness she was not the best historian and it was difficult to get a clear history as to the nature of the incontinence, direct questioning usually resulting in some form of affirmative response. She complained primarily of waking up wet at night. She had taken to wearing nappies and these were always soaked by the morning. She explained that she went to the toilet frequently and could not hold her urine for long if she was delayed. She voided small quantities at these times. She also leaked small quantities of urine on coughing or straining when she was unprepared for activity. She was uncertain as to the duration of her symptoms but they had been present for many years. She had no discomfort before, during or after the passage of urine. The urine was not unusually offensive. There was no haematuria.

The patient was known to have a hiatus hernia for which she took cimetidine. A solitary gallstone had been identified during the investigation of her dyspepsia but as her symptoms had resolved on medication this was not pursued further. She was on no other medication.

Nine years before she had complained to her GP about a prolapse. This she had tolerated since the birth of her daughter some 40 years earlier. This had been easily reducible until 3 years before when it became more difficult to do so. She needed to reduce the uterus digitally before she could pass urine properly. She complained then of occasional dysuria and frequency of micturition at night but there was no incontinence. She had been admitted to hospital and had undergone surgery. The plan had been to remove the uterus but on recovery she was told that it had been 'hitched up'. Initially everything had gone well but 6 months after the operation her prolapse returned and then gradually the incontinence developed.

On examination she was well orientated and communicative. She weighed 70.3 kg. Her BP was 150/90 mmHg and examination of the cardiorespiratory system was normal. The abdomen was obese but not distended. There was no organomegaly and the hernial orifices were intact. There was a prominent midline subumbilical scar. There was no incisional hernia.

On vaginal examination there was an obvious total procidentia. The dependent cervix was hypertrophied and cornified but there was no ulceration. The uterus reduced easily into the vagina. The perineum was very deficient. On bimanual examination the uterus was not unduly enlarged although the cervix was elongated. There were no pelvic masses. With the uterus reduced coughing resulted in the loss of a small quantity of urine. This could be prevented by the digital elevation of the urethrovesical angle. The vagina was voluminous and there were no scars from previous surgery.

After her attendance at hospital temporary relief of the prolapse was attempted by using a ring pessary but this was soon expelled. Larger rings and a shelf pessary failed to control the prolapse.

What is your assessment of this case?

This elderly patient presents with a procidentia and a history of incontinence. The history is suggestive of bladder irritability but the findings on examination would support a dimension of sphincter incompetence. The picture is complicated by the history of an earlier operation the true nature of which is obscure but which appears to have been a purely abdominal procedure.

How would you proceed?

I would set about determining her suitability for surgery as she is clearly limited by her symptoms and simple measures have failed. Blood should be obtained for haemoglobin and plasma urea and electrolytes. She requires a chest X-ray and ECG and a midstream specimen of urine should be sent for microscopy, culture and sensitivity. The history is of a long-standing prolapse and incontinence. The upper renal tract might be damaged and an IVU is indicated.

The nature of her first operation could limit the options for surgery this time. I would write to request details of the last operation.

The exact nature of her incontinence is obscure and in part this is made more difficult by the patient's difficulty in clearly describing her symptoms, no matter how carefully questions are put to her. I would request a full cystometric evaluation of her bladder function.

The tests you selected to determine her suitability for surgery were all satisfactory. The previous notes explain that when assessed 9 years ago it was only possible to partially reduce the uterus because of a stony hard irregular mass filling the left side of the pelvis and which was fixed. An X-ray confirmed a large calcified fibroid. Arrangements were made for her to be admitted initially for myomectomy to be followed at a later date by a vaginal hysterectomy and pelvic floor repair. At operation a calcified fibroid the size of a fetal head was removed from the left and posterior wall of the uterus. The fibroid, weighing 850 g, was removed after dissection off the back of the uterus. Both ovaries were removed. The peritoneum was closed around the uterus the fundus 'being exteriorized into the rectus sheath'. The uterus was fixed to the rectus sheath with nylon. The ultrasound examination confirmed a normal urinary tract and no significant residual urine in the bladder after voiding.

How does this information affect your management?

The description of her previous operation rules out a vaginal hysterectomy as an option to control her prolapse. Although the uterus is small and freely mobile there is no knowing the situation within the abdomen concerning adhesions and attachments to other structures. The last operation appears to have been a strictly extempore procedure.

An abdominal procedure is essential to resolve the prolapse satisfactorily although a Le Fort colpocleisis would be an alternative to avoid a possibly difficult abdominal procedure if the problem were simply one of prolapse. This lady is very fit for her age and should tolerate a major procedure well. The selection as to which operation to advise will depend upon the findings on cystometry.

The cystometry report showed that the bladder was stable to a capacity of 350 ml. There was no evidence of uninhibited bladder activity on filling or on provocation. The voiding occurred by a combination of straining and detrusor contraction and a peak flow was only 5 ml/s. She felt this was slow for her as she achieved a better stream when she reduced her prolapse before voiding. On reducing her prolapse genuine stress incontinence was demonstrable.

This patient's surgical management presents something of a problem. In view of her previous surgery a vaginal approach might entail considerable risk. The best approach to her prolapse might be an abdominal hysterectomy with colposacropexy. The latter should prevent the risk of a subsequent vault prolapse as the tissues are so very poor. The concern about this approach is that on reducing her prolapse her stress incontinence becomes more of a problem. A way forward would be to incorporate a colposuspension into the procedure. Even so having thus straightened out her bladder base there would be some risk of postoperative voiding dysfunction. The poor flow rate is not reassuring. Considering the severity of her various problems a total abdominal hysterectomy colposuspension and colposacropexy would seem to be the operation of choice. The situation needs to be discussed thoroughly with the patient. If a voiding difficulty were to persist after surgery then clean intermittent self catheterization might be necessary.

Discussion

It is a fact that some gynaecologists are more enthusiastic about vaginal surgery than others. This particularly relates to the vaginal hysterectomy. Some advocates would maintain that it is possible to perform a vaginal hysterectomy in the absence of prolapse providing that there were no specific contraindications in terms of associated pathology. Others would ask 'Why do a difficult vaginal operation when a straightforward abdominal procedure would suffice'? There is general agreement however that the vaginal approach to hysterectomy is better when dealing with prolapse or vaginal laxity. Even here there may be some contradictions from those who enthuse about the Manchester procedure.

It is difficult to make an objective assessment about the relative merits of vaginal as opposed to abdominal hysterectomy because the former is not undertaken in the presence of severe pelvic disease or if the uterus is considerably enlarged. Likewise the morbidity of a vaginal hysterectomy combined with an extensive anterior and posterior repair may well be greater than for an abdominal procedure to remove the uterus and adnexae for a simple myoma. Where comparable series have been reported it has been observed that the operating time for the vaginal hysterectomy is shorter. However it is not possible to perform a laparotomy via this route and the unexpected discovery of enlarged ovaries can pose a problem. The total blood loss for a vaginal procedure is less but where the indications are comparable the losses for abdominal procedures are not excessive. There is little doubt that the mobilization and convalescence of the vaginal hysterectomy patient is much smoother without the discomfort of an abdominal wound. Postoperative fever is reported more commonly for vaginal hysterectomy although the incidence of demonstrable infection is higher for the abdominal approach. Paralytic ileus, peritonitis, respiratory infection, venous thrombosis and pulmonary embolism are all possible after vaginal hysterectomy but are commoner after the abdominal approach. It should be remembered, however, that figures quoted usually refer to all hysterectomies including the difficult ones not suitable for a vaginal procedure. Even so, the operative mortality for the abdominal approach is three times that of the vaginal operation, despite the latter being undertaken more frequently on the older patient.

Comment

It is not always possible to get a clear lucid history from a patient. If the candidate encounters trouble in this respect then certainly it should be referred to in the presentation of the history. The history here was bizarre, but the examiner purposely kept the discussion within the compass of the candidate. It is important not to panic when faced with the unexpected or unusual. What does matter is the clear presentation of the history, the careful demonstration of any physical signs and an orderly assessment of the case leading to a reasonable programme for management on the information available.

Further reading

COPENHAVER, E. H. (1965) Hysterectomy: Vaginal versus Abdominal. *Surgical Clinics of North America*, **45**, 751–763

Appendix 1

Crown rump length (CRL) v gestational age (25,50,75 centiles)

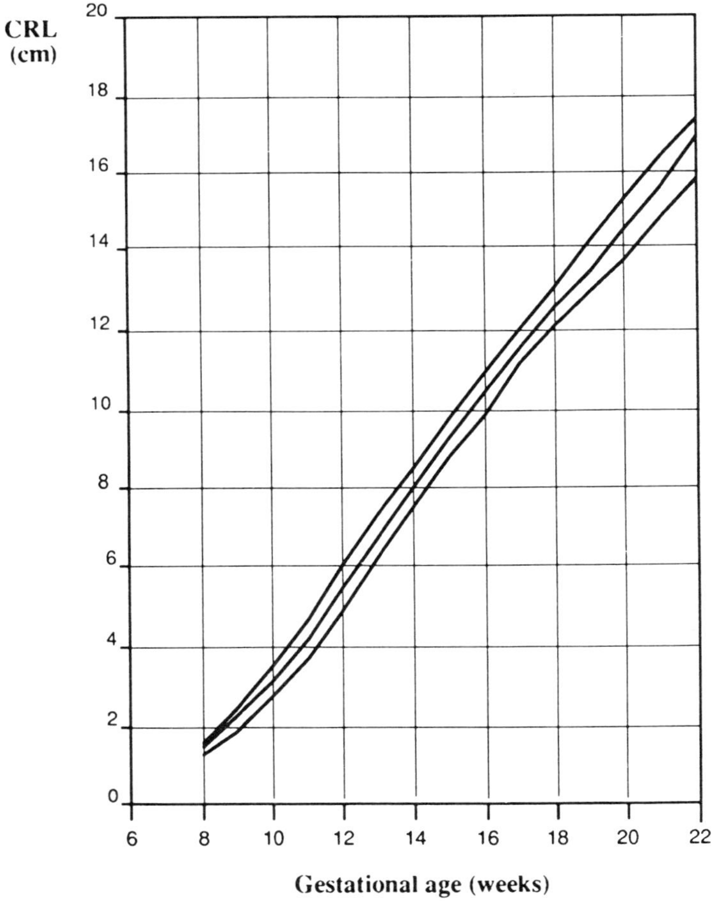

Appendix 2

Biparietal diameter v gestational age (mean ± 2SD)

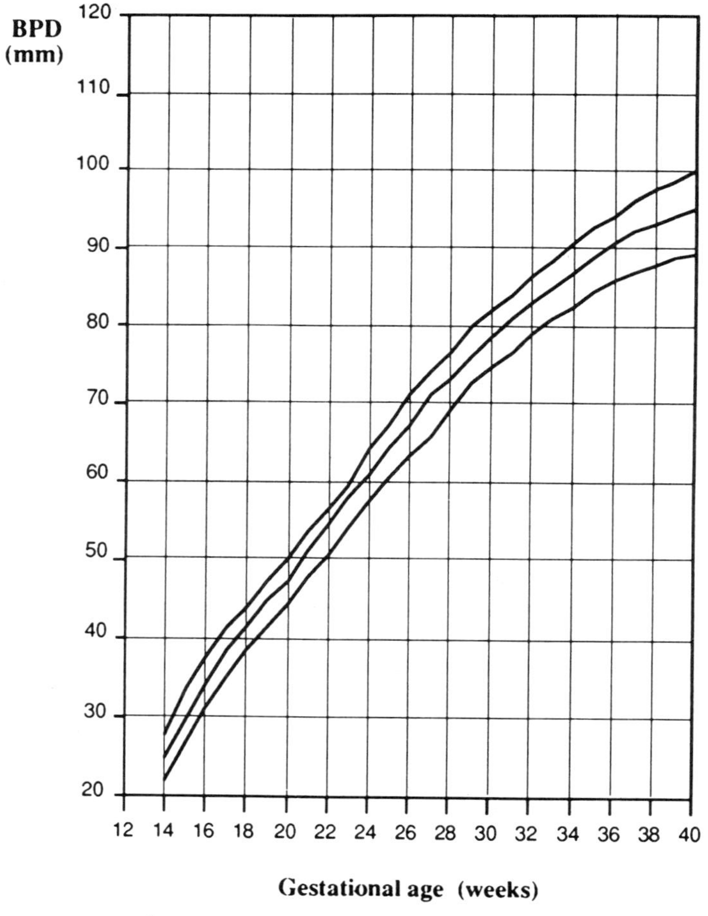

Appendix 3

Head circumference (HC) and abdominal circumference (AC) v gestational age (mean ± 2SD)

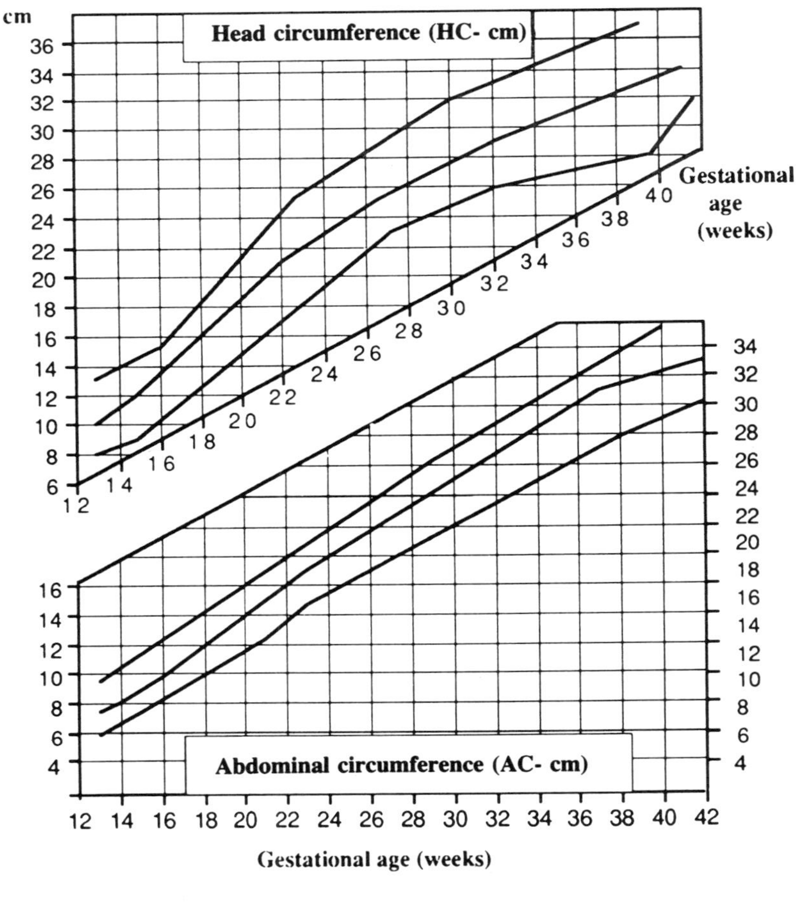

Appendix 4

Relation between gestational age and birthweight

Singleton pregnancies, 5th, mean & 95th centiles, not corrected for sex

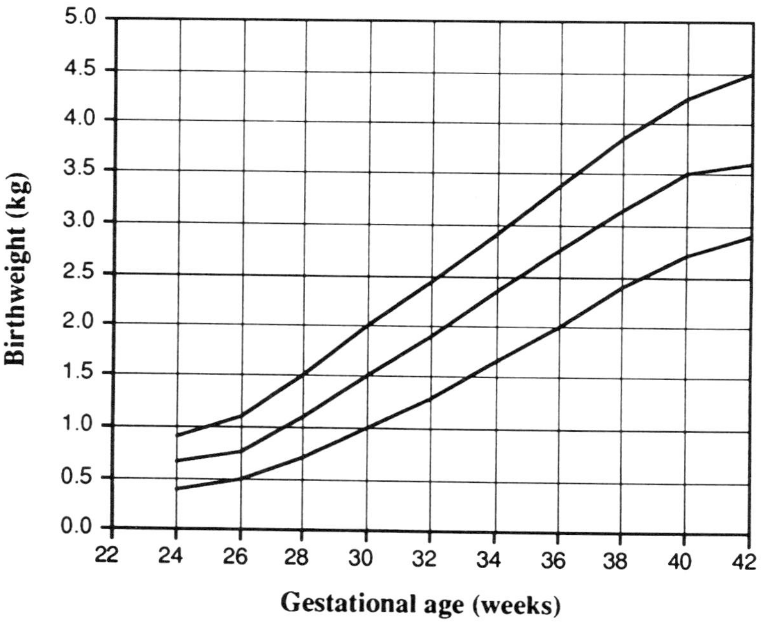

Appendix 5

Normal adult values

Plasma hormone levels

LH	Follicular phase:	1–6 U/l
	Mid cycle:	up to 25 U/l
	Luteal phase:	1–3 U/l
FSH	Follicular phase:	1–8 U/l
	Mid cycle:	up to 15 U/l
	Luteal phase:	0.5–3 U/l
Prolactin:		< 450 mU/l
17-beta-oestradiol	Follicular phase:	70–370 pmol/l
	Luteal phase:	90–870 pmol/l
Progesterone:	Follicular phase:	< 5 nmol/l
	Luteal phase:	> 20 nmol/l
Testosterone:		< 3.1 nmol/l
Sex hormone binding globulin (SHBG):		20–95 mmol/l
Androstenedione:		< 12 nmol/l
17-alpha-hydroxyprogesterone:		< 14 nmol/l
Dehydroepiandrosterone:		8.3–46.7 nmol/l
Dehydroepiandrosterone sulphate:		0.8–9.3 μmol/l
Cortisol (09.00):		190–720 nmol/l
(24.00):		< 220 nmol/l
Thyroxine (T4):		63–131 nmol/l
Free thyroxine index:		21–36
Tri-iodothyronine:		1.2–3.0 nmol/l
TSH:		1–6 mmol/l
Glycosylated haemoglobin (HbA1c):		5–7.5%
Fasting insulin:		2.8–13.5 mU/l
Glucose:		3.3–5.0 mmol/l

Serum values

Sodium:	136–142 mmol/l
Potassium:	3.4–4.4 mmol/l
Chloride:	100–108 mmol/l
Bicarbonate:	25–32 mmol/l
Urea:	2.8–7.7 mmol/l
Creatinine:	61–125 μmol/l
Bilirubin:	3–21 μmol/l
Aspartate transaminase:	< 37 U/l
Gamma-glutamyltransaminase:	< 40 U/l
Total protein:	62–79 g/l
Albumin:	39–51 g/l

Index